The Anxiety
Reset Method

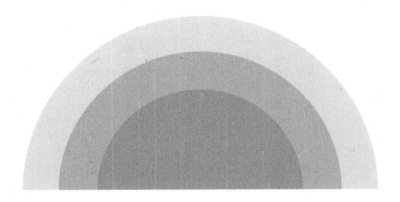

The Anxiety Reset Method

Master Your Anxious Mind in 12 Weeks

Georgie Collinson

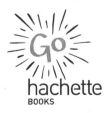

hachette
BOOKS

New York

Hachette Go, an imprint of Hachette Books
Hachette Book Group
1290 Avenue of the Americas
New York, NY 10104
HachetteGo.com
Facebook.com/HachetteGo
Instagram.com/HachetteGo

First US Edition: October 2023

Published by Hachette Go, an imprint of Hachette Book Group, Inc. The Hachette Go name and logo are trademarks of the Hachette Book Group.

The Hachette Speakers Bureau provides a wide range of authors for speaking events. To find out more, go to hachettespeakersbureau.com or email HachetteSpeakers@hbgusa.com.

Hachette Go books may be purchased in bulk for business, educational, or promotional use. For information, please contact your local bookseller or email the Hachette Book Group Special Markets Department at Special.Markets@hbgusa.com.

The publisher is not responsible for websites (or their content) that are not owned by the publisher.

Library of Congress Cataloging-in-Publication Data

Name: Collinson, Georgie, author.
Title: The anxiety reset method: master your anxious mind in 12 weeks / Georgie Collinson.
Description: New York: Go, Hachette Books, 2023. |
    Includes bibliographical references.
Identifiers: LCCN 2023027375 | ISBN 9780306834783 (paper over board) |
    ISBN 9780306834790 (ebook)
Subjects: LCSH: Anxiety. | Self-help techniques.
Classification: LCC BF575.A6 C65 2023 | DDC 152.4/6—dc23/eng/20230626
LC record available at https://lccn.loc.gov/2023027375

ISBNs: 978-0-306-83478-3 (paper over board); 978-0-306-83479-0 (ebook)

Printed in the United States of America

LSC-C

Printing 1, 2023

For my late grandmother, Lois, whose vivacious spirit and unconditional love mirror the true self within.

Contents

Author's Note

The information in this book does not constitute medical advice. It is for informational purposes only, and it is not intended to diagnose, treat, cure, or prevent any condition or disease. Diagnosis and treatment of any mental health condition requires the attention of a physician or qualified mental health professional. Please consult your healthcare provider before applying any of the information, to ensure the advice is right for you. Any case studies are composites of real clients, whose names and details have been changed to protect their privacy. Although I have used certain gendered terms in this book, such as male and female hormones and masculine and feminine energies, I have done so for concision, and those gendered elements can apply to anyone. And finally, this book has been written to include everyone, with regard to gender, sexuality, and race, and it is my hope that every reader can relate to the examples included.

Introduction

When I meet someone new and they discover I help people with high-functioning anxiety, very often they respond, "Oh god, that's me. I need you!" If this is you too, you're not alone.

High-functioning anxiety is the perfectionistic, pressure-fueled type where, despite the anxious feelings, day-to-day activities are accomplished and generally well-executed. It's a common experience for many high achievers. Being perfect and working as hard as you can is pretty much embedded in society's values. But the fact that this behavior is normalized doesn't mean it's good for us, or that we can't change it.

Sometimes I try to imagine all the people across the world experiencing high-functioning anxiety, and it feels incredibly overwhelming. I think they deserve so much better. In choosing to pick up this book, it is quite likely you're one of those people. When I picture you opening up to the first page and finding these words, I can't help but beam with excitement for you. I know that the possibility of a new life awaits.

Maybe you're exhausted. Maybe you're tired of being at war with yourself in your quest to be perfect all the time. Maybe you're weary from looking to other people to give you the love you crave. Maybe you have no idea what you're really meant to be doing with your life. Maybe you yearn for your relationships to feel more connected.

Maybe your heart feels battered and scarred from life's disappointments. Maybe you've started to develop health issues that won't go away. Maybe you're done with putting everyone else first and leaving yourself last. Maybe your wildest dreams and deepest heart's desires feel way out of reach.

Maybe you're feeling like you never have enough: not enough time, money, friends, praise, love. Maybe you're over making other people happy and caring so much about what they think of you. Maybe your inner critic is yelling loudly, pulling you apart piece by piece every time you look in the mirror. Maybe, more days than you'd like to admit, the voice of self-doubt is all you can hear.

If you find yourself repeating habits that don't really serve you, you might find answers in these pages. Numbing ourselves from uncomfortable emotions and not knowing how to stop is very common, and it's something I've experienced myself. So many of us have a lot of great things going on, but our lives don't really make us happy in the way society promises. Often, something about our life just feels off, but we can't quite put our finger on it. If you're curious about the possibility of something other than the hamster-wheel way of life, living with your anxious mind controlling you, I'm so happy you picked up this book.

I know what it's like to feel like you can't trust life enough to let go and enjoy the ride. I too have lived from that fearful place, armored up with tension in my neck and shoulders. I know how it feels to be hyperaware of what others think and to have a mind consumed with circling worries that promise to keep you safe in the world—and hold you back from living freely from your heart.

If you're not sure what living from your heart is just yet, don't worry: We'll work on that. It's enough right now to know it's about that niggle you feel, calling you to something new, luring you toward a different solution. It's that tiny glimmer of hope you catch yourself letting in sometimes, that inner excitement and sense of joy that bubbles up spontaneously within you. Maybe that feeling seems like a distant memory, but it's there, and it's enough to get you started.

I wrote this book for those in a similar place to where I once was—to give you hope that you *can* take positive action toward creating a life full of joy and power. You *can* become the master of your anxious mind. I've helped thousands of people claim this kind of power for themselves, and it's there for the taking for you too.

That said, this is not a book about "curing" or "fixing" anxiety. I know you wish you could just get rid of your anxiety and the discomfort that comes with it—but the key is to change how you relate to anxiety altogether. Anxiety is not something you actually *want* to remove from your life experience. Let me explain.

The "eradicate anxiety" approach just doesn't work. The more you try to silence it, the louder anxiety will roar back in response. It's a fickle creature, much like a cat who refuses to be affectionate when you want him to be. The cat, in defiance, will jump away from your outstretched fingers. At that point, many people give up and say cats are too difficult to deal with. People say that about anxiety too, after just a few attempts to make it better. The cat will come to you purring when you learn to understand how he operates and how to work with his rules and temperament. You must learn to approach the cat the way he wants you to: just after he has woken from a nap, ready for a scratch under the chin. Anxiety works in much the same way.

We have to learn how to take the "wrongness" out of anxiety. This intense emotional state is not a tumor to cut out, it's a compass pointing to where you can grow, find more love within, and build the kind of self-confidence that has you calling in whatever you wish your life to be. Anxiety is the loud noise you hear when your car veers over the guiding white lines on the highway of your life. Anxiety says, "Hey, you might want to adjust the wheel a little. Don't keep going this way!" Instead of trying to shut it down, approach anxiety with curiosity. See the value it can offer in your life: the fuel for transformative growth it provides and the important messages hidden within its discomfort. Appreciate the way it signals the need for more sleep, better nutrition, and taking care of your physical body.

We must learn to see beyond the fears and limits of the anxious mind to find our true nature beneath. Our true nature is trusting the journey of life, no matter how uncertain the path ahead may seem. Our true nature is feeling comfortable and alive in our bodies. Our true nature is feeling safe and expansive, like life is full of opportunities and possibilities. Our true nature is loving the human beings around us with compassion and without judgment. Most importantly, our true nature is loving ourselves. It's navigating life's challenges with the ability to switch out of fear and into self-love that gives you the best outcome. This is mastering your anxious mind.

I will soon share the details of my story and how I learned to reset my anxious mind, but because I am sure you'll want to know this part right away, let me fast-forward to the end and assure you that, these days, anxiety has no power over me. I know just what to do when anxiety shows up (and it still does from time to time). The crucial difference is that the anxiety passes on through quietly, taking up little of my energy or brain space. I have no interest in the fear-mongering stories it offers up and do not pay attention to its doubts or judgments. All that energy is now available for investing in important relationships, putting my health first, dreaming up new projects, showing up in my business, painting and singing, traveling the world, helping others, following my heart's desires, and prioritizing what truly matters in life.

This expansive, openhearted way of living is available to you too if you will agree to one rule: Your aim is *not* to never feel anxious again. You must not beat yourself up when you're feeling anxious yet again. That is another sneaky way for perfectionism to block you from the growth and healing you're seeking. If you commit yourself to following my instructions, you will reach a place where you experience much less anxiety much less of the time, but you haven't failed if you feel moments of anxiety all through your life. As I said, I still feel anxiety sometimes too. The most important question to ask is: Did you respond differently in that moment of anxiety?

You will feel anxious at times as you move through the healing process of this book. Please expect that and know that you will be okay. I will guide you through these anxious moments as we go. The truth is, you have so much more power over anxiety than you realize. Healing is a process of recognizing that power and stepping into it more and more—then losing it, then finding it again. Such is the journey of our lives. There is no fairy-tale story in which the caterpillar goes into a healing cocoon and emerges as a butterfly and that's it: It lives happily ever after with no challenges or pain. You're never done. You will go back into the cocoon and be forced to find your wings again and again. It can feel grueling at times, but remember that the healing process is oh so beautiful too. Each time you will emerge wiser, stronger, and, if you embrace your healing, more at peace with what life is all about. When you realize there is no mountain peak to aim for, you become a lot more accepting of the process and content with where you are along the way. That acceptance makes the journey so much easier, as anxiety has nothing to cling to. The ins and outs of practicing this art will all come later. For now, please believe me that you are not truly the anxious, highly strung person you think you are. You are so much more than that, and together we'll prove this.

I understand that you've probably been seeking answers and searching for a better way of life for a long time. I've been there. Once upon a time, all I could see in my future was a black hole. It was like a vague impending doom, and I had to prepare for it. I was just waiting for the next big world-shaking moment to come and get me. I tried a few psychologists but I never found the right one for me. I didn't walk away with tools I could readily use or the deep transformation I desired. I tried supporting myself through nutrition. I thought if I just ate all the right foods my brain would function differently and the anxiety would go away. But I went overboard with rules and restrictions, and the anxiety got worse. I threw all my hopes into healing my gut, somehow expecting my life to fall into place. Gut health is important but, on its own, it didn't have a big impact. These silver-bullet solutions are alluring, but only considering one piece of the puzzle is bound to end in disappointment. We must look at all of anxiety's intricate parts.

Understanding and teaching the components that make up a calm, confident, and resilient life has become my life's work. I developed the Anxiety Reset Method as a way to bring all these components together into a holistic system that actually works. This approach considers the impact of your thoughts, food, gut health, hormones, and the way you live your daily life. It's about leaving no stone unturned as you empower yourself to grow beyond anxiety.

Bringing people out of that fearful, limited, stressed-out state and back into their hearts with their arms stretched open to all that life has to offer is the most rewarding part of the work I do. The world needs more beautiful people like you living bravely from their hearts, don't you think?

How to Use This Book

Mastery Is the Goal

To master your anxious mind, you must understand how the mind works and use that awareness to empower yourself and choose your experience. Anxiety can't survive for long when you have the knowledge, tools, and skills to see through the mind's lies and tricks, tempting you back into fear, time after time.

True mind mastery is a process of learning to live in awareness, then forgetting and returning to unconsciousness, before catching yourself and coming back to awareness, over and over. It's making the choice to see the gaps in your resilience (because you're human!) and build upon them. It's asking the anxiety what it is trying to tell you and lovingly offering yourself what you need in response.

When you practice mastering your anxious mind, you will feel a sense of confidence and stability deep within you that no one can take from you. The challenges you face will only serve to strengthen your ability to overcome anything that comes your way—because you know that you can find a way to feel powerful in your life, no matter what.

A Holistic Road Map for Anxiety

The Anxiety Reset Method combines a variety of modalities I have collected over the years to create a unique healing experience. I'm an anxiety mindset coach, hypnotherapist, and degree-qualified nutritionist and naturopath. It has been my privilege to work with clients around the world, addressing high-functioning anxiety from a holistic perspective, and watch them flourish as a result.

The method we'll work through in this book covers all the factors that lead to high-functioning anxiety—from addressing your mindset and beliefs to taking care of your physical body. You can follow it as a blueprint for your own growth and self-development. If you have the determination required to apply these tools in your life, you will be guided back home to your true self—beneath the pressure, perfectionism, and exhausting critique from the anxious mind that you currently feel controls you.

I wrote the book intending you to work through the Anxiety Reset Method week by week in a linear fashion; after reading the whole way through, you might like to return to a certain chapter or even open a page at random when you need a quick hit of guidance and support.

Before we begin, some recommendations for you:

- **Keep a journal:** Have a notebook nearby and a place to write and reflect in response to the questions and exercises in this book. Avoid using a screen for this purpose. Putting pen to paper has therapeutic benefits in itself, so I really encourage you to go low tech with this.
- **Make time to practice:** The practices within each chapter are your weekly action steps. The detailed instructions for the work required can be found within the chapters. Reading this

book is one thing, but actually implementing the action steps is another. If you really want to change, you must take action. To take action, you must dedicate some space in your life for it. The time you spend on each practice will vary. Schedule in a dedicated hour each week to allow for the practices and approach this as nurturing, restful time in your week for you to reconnect with yourself. Many people who have been through my online program find Sunday mornings or afternoons work well. There's also a checklist at the end of each chapter you can tick off once you've completed the work.

- **Take mental notes:** As you work through each week's chapter, you'll encounter sections titled Mental Notes. Mental Notes are quick reminders of important points you may like to revisit. These key concepts have been particularly helpful to my program members. They're the ideas I often remind them to revisit. I invite you to write your own Mental Notes too, and copy into your journal any of mine that resonate.

- **Take a news break:** I encourage you to cancel or unsubscribe from any news sources and avoid news programs during your time working through this material. Delete any news apps that send you notifications throughout the day. The news and media can fuel our worries, anxieties, and concerns in a way that does not serve us much of the time. We see a skewed version of reality and the world, with emphasis on negativity. We hear about shocking events happening on the other side of the world that we can't do anything about. We feel powerless. It does take its toll on your mental health. If you've never taken a break from the news before, I encourage you to make the most of this opportunity to see how you feel. If something important happens in the world, trust me, you will hear about it. Peace and clarity come when we're not seeking this kind of information more than is necessary. Remember, this time of transformation is all about you—not the external world or anyone else.

Now Is the Time to Start

You can always find excuses not to do this work. There will always be problems in your life that make it feel like now is not the right time. Your mind is an expert at finding these problems. It will pretty much always be a "bad time" to start doing the inner work. The elusive, perfect, peaceful time to get this done doesn't exist. Actually, most people find that the support I provide in my online program, upon which this book is based, makes the big life challenges a whole lot easier to manage as they go through them. But if you don't apply what I have to teach you and commit to this work, you simply won't get results.

This is a gentle wake-up call to no longer let the problems in your life and the world put you off. This is your opportunity to just start, wherever you are, no matter how messy it all looks. Take that one step forward in the mud, and the next, and the next after that. This process has been designed with busy people in mind, so the exercises should not take hours and hours out of your week. Over time, these subtle adjustments simply become woven into the way you live your life, so that every day you are reinforcing your own anxiety resilience.

It's Going to Get Uncomfortable

Now it's time for a loving reality check. If you want to make progress and stop feeling so out of control with stress and anxiety, you must be prepared to invite some discomfort into your life. This work isn't for the fainthearted. All that determination that you so readily channel into your career, family, or relationship is going to come in handy here. It requires you to be ready to look at the parts of yourself that you haven't wanted to look at. It asks you to question things you haven't wanted to question. It politely requests that you get curious and make space for feelings you haven't wanted to feel. It extends an invitation for you to really get to know yourself intimately, so you can feel a whole lot better.

If this idea makes you cringe, be mindful that you're already uncomfortable in the anxiety and self-doubt cycle. There's plenty of discomfort in your life, but right now you feel you have no power or choice around it. That's as uncomfortable as it gets. This book asks you to consciously choose the flavor of discomfort you want to experience—which is so much better than just being uncomfortable, stuck, and powerless. Leaning into your chosen discomfort of exploring and testing out new, unfamiliar ways of relating to anxiety will bring the biggest rewards. That's certainly what I discovered after the years I spent trying anything to avoid feeling uncomfortable.

Anxiety in My Life

From Rock to Quicksand

When I was nineteen years old I was pretty sure I had the best family. The five of us were a solid rock I could depend on so deeply that I didn't really think much about it. My family unit was always there. We all still lived at home together then. My dad used to make me laugh with his odd declarations as he arrived home after work, booming "I am the man" as he walked through the front door. We used to joke that he'd never function in the world without Mom. She'd pack his suitcase for him, have dinner ready every night, lay out supplements for him to take each morning, and sort out all the essential tasks that kept life running behind the scenes. He was a loyal man, but work was always his priority. He even had his office set up so he could sleep there if he needed to. Apart from work, we made up the rest of his world. My mom has a heart of gold and she was the quintessential self-sacrificing mother to us kids. I was very close with my siblings. My brother was my best friend and my sister and I would play around with the guitar together, singing harmonies from our favorite musicals. I was the youngest, and as true as the stereotype goes, I really did get away with murder. Innocent little me was the last to blame for every sibling spat, and I always believed I was Dad's favorite.

In July of that year, two months after my nineteenth birthday, we took our last family holiday together. My siblings and I were making jokes by the pool while a few meters away, in an air-conditioned hotel room safe from the thick Bali heat, our parents were having a very different conversation. Dad told Mom he was having an affair with another woman—a woman so much younger that she was just two years older than my sister.

Mom couldn't hide her distress from me and my sister as the three of us window-shopped on the way to have dinner as a family that night. Our questioning became impossible to dodge. In our family there were few secrets. Keeping private information to yourself was considered highly suspicious, almost to the point of absurd. When Mom finally unloaded what Dad had said to her, we could hardly believe her. This didn't make any sense. No, Dad needed Mom. If anything, we always thought Mom might leave him. My whole reality tore in two. I remember the numbness and the rapid, sweet wash of denial. It was so easy in those first few moments to pretend like nothing had happened at all. Eyes fixed on my feet as I walked along the dusty road, I took solace in the idea that maybe it was all a bad dream.

But the bad dream never ended. Dad flew home early without us. We were left to dwell in the suffocating humidity of that tropical paradise horror movie for a few days longer. And, just like that, my heart broke properly for the first time.

Dad moved out of the family home within a week. My rock turned to quicksand and the sinking feeling stayed much too long. Though Dad said his decision had nothing to do with me, it didn't feel that way. My whole concept of the kind of man he was had been crumpled up like paper and torn into bits. There was loyal, respectable, silly old Dad, and now this other person, this vile stranger I did not know. A man who would cut his family up into fragments. Through this experience, I faced a hard truth we must all eventually come to learn as we go through life: that certainty is a myth. Nothing is certain and everything changes. It's a pretty messed-up game, this life, hey?

In the days, weeks, and months that followed I was all too aware of the shaky ground upon which I stood. Life somersaulted into a battleground, gray and bleak. During my high school years I had experienced a fair bit of anxiety when it came to impressing boys, feeling insecure about my body, and getting good grades. My inner critic and perfectionism were already well matured. But now, anxiety unlike any I'd ever experienced before had awoken within me. It had a beastly fervor to it. I wasn't naive anymore. I'd grown wiser. I knew the next shock in life would come for me again. I now found myself ducking for cover from mind-made fear bombs. Someone I love could die, or maybe I'd run out of money, or what if I never found peace in my life ever again? I couldn't exactly name the disaster scenario heading for me in much detail, but something was coming. Something bad. And I had to prepare, just in case. I wasn't completely aware of it at the time, but looking back, I see how a strong urge to fight the uncertainty grew within me. I needed to create some kind of stability in the chaos. That was the only way I could survive.

What could I do to create stability? Well, that part wasn't so clear. But the anxiety that woke me every morning to remind me how my life had gone terribly wrong was certainly willing to try. I came up with plan after plan.

Maybe I could find it in the perfect diet, the anxiety suggested. So I tried that. I read all the nutrition books and pored over recipe blogs written by naturally thin women in bikinis. I tested out going vegan, keto, paleo, and everything in between. I even decided to study nutrition and naturopathy, a passion that was in all honesty initially driven by my desire to be perfect. Because maybe if I ate perfectly enough, I'd have the perfect body. And with the perfect body, I'd feel more confident in myself—more desirable and worthy. Maybe that would give me a sense of safety. Maybe that would ease this restless, uncomfortable buzzing feeling. (Spoiler alert: it didn't.)

As I continued my studies, I learned that nutrition could increase the calming chemicals in my brain so I'd be more resilient to life's challenges. This was a convenient way to convince myself and others that I was drinking the green smoothie sludge (more an unappealing brown color in those days) for my mental and physical health. "It's not a diet. It's a lifestyle," I'd tell people.

But really, if I was honest with myself, I wanted the perfect body. Like many others I had been seduced by the belief that if I could just eat all the "right" foods, life would be wonderful. Acai-eating Instagram influencers—the perfect smiling models and famous wellness gurus I looked up to—assured me this dream could come true for me. The perfect body promised me happiness and love, and surely there's no better way to create certainty than that.

I had a big list of things I couldn't eat. I'd cringe if family members or friends offered me certain food ingredients I'd labeled "the devil." There was no fooling my brain that my food rules were a lifestyle rather than a diet. My brain responded the way brains are wired to respond to restrictive diets. On the way home from nutrition lectures, I'd find myself binge-eating packs of pricey vegan chocolate in my car, hiding the rubbish in the public bin before walking into the house. I'd go to bed at night feeling like a failure, swearing I just needed more willpower. The anxiety only grew louder.

"Maybe certainty can be found in a relationship," the anxiety offered. "If he never leaves you, that will make up for the horrible pain you feel because your dad left. You'll have someone who'll always love you, and that will make you happy." So I made sure that I chose a partner who wouldn't leave me, one I could trust and who thought the world of me. But then the anxiety worried that I was missing out on lots of exciting things in life by being in a safe relationship and I needed to have more experiences to make the most of my precious life (and relentless clock-ticking youth). At first it was a whisper, but soon the anxious mind started to yell at me: "What if you're not making the most of your twenties? What if you regret the way you're spending these years?" As time went on, I found myself more frequently in tears on the bedroom floor—brick-wall stuck, sad, and anxious. Somehow I was now unraveling the carefully woven stability I'd been creating with my partner, pulling it all apart, thread by thread. I berated myself for it. It didn't make any sense, and it was clear that I still wasn't happy. I didn't like who I was. I didn't like my life. And nothing about that felt stable.

"Maybe it's in having enough money," the anxiety tried next. "With money, you can travel all the time and have lots of exciting things happening so that you never need to face the bleakness of the battleground or the reality of uncertainty. You can have a nice life, buy pretty clothes, and feel free to do whatever you want." Soon enough, my goal to build a career or start a business with a brilliant idea became an obsession that anxiety loved to stew on. Financial security was the green light at the end of the dock that I yearned for but never seemed to reach. It was never enough. I was never there. It didn't matter how much my bank account grew or stagnated or how many steps forward I made in my journey. And so, my relentless search for a way out of anxiety continued.

Unshakable Composure

Since that time I've found solace in seeing that no matter how winding the road, somehow we are always on the right path. Eventually the dots join up, even when it feels so offtrack at the time. Looking back it appears as though my life slotted into place easily, as if I'd planned it. I couldn't have felt further from a plan as I navigated my way through the muck, searching for a way to feel good in myself and calm my gnawing anxious mind.

My unhealthy relationship with food didn't help me find the answers right away, but I am grateful it led me to study nutrition and naturopathy. My four-year degree was only the start, ultimately the foundation of developing the Anxiety Reset Method. I learned about nutrition, gut health, hormones, herbal medicine, and how to discern between quality research and sloppy studies that don't hold much power in the science world. I did a lot of good things for my body during this time too. I worked on all aspects of my health, from my hormones to my gut health. I stopped taking the oral contraceptive pill and learned to track, understand, and find flow in my life with the seasons of my natural cycles. I started adding greens to my breakfast, stayed away from caffeine, and took shots of apple cider vinegar each morning. I learned to base my meals around plenty of protein and incorporated a few key guidelines I will teach you later in this book.

Nutrition started to feel like a language I could speak fluently, without much mental effort. As I worked deeply with my emotions, beliefs, and mindset, my rules with food eased, and I started to see food as fuel for my body again. Through such practices as I'll guide you through in this book, I began building my physiological resilience to anxiety. With my brain receiving more nutrients I could think calmly and clearly. As I became more nourished and resilient, anxiety visited less frequently. However, as I mentioned, working on the physical elements related to anxiety weren't the complete answer for me either.

The other aspect of my healing was a little more complex, bridging the scientific and the spiritual. I had to figure out how to build a deep sense of trust in life. I had to learn about the inner workings of the mind. I needed to question what I believed and rewire the habitual thought patterns that drove my fear. I did a lot of the work by myself, and you can too. I also worked with healers and coaches, and I very much encourage you to bring others on board if that helps you feel more supported. An outside perspective is invaluable for shifting deep-seated beliefs. Let me make one thing clear, though: As brilliant as it would be for someone to wave a magic wand over you and fix your problems, healing is not something another person can do for you. You must be fully open to the process and choose it for yourself. Healing requires ongoing work.

As I hope I've made abundantly clear, I wasn't always a positive person. Who I am now is the person I have crafted myself into, and I did this deliberately. I used the same resolve that once had me cramming all night for an exam or starving my body on a three-day juice cleanse, albeit this time with a much more self-loving undertone. You can make this choice for yourself, to love yourself as hard as you've worked on something else in your life. If you've read this far in, chances are you've already started.

I learned many techniques along the way. My journal played a major role too. As I mentioned previously, I did try traditional psychotherapy, but I wasn't able to find a psychologist I clicked with or who took me to the depths I was willing to go to (though this is not necessarily everyone's experience). This had me looking elsewhere, searching out other solutions beyond the mainstream. It's why in my coaching work today I can offer a different approach for those on a path more like mine, for those who feel called to seek something more. Hopeful curiosity and my determination that my early experiences would not be my life story carried me through my healing. (You have this ability in you too.) I moved forward, step-by-step, asking different questions, fueled by the belief that something out there had to help me.

And then it found me. You know how sometimes you hear the right message at the right time and it strikes a chord with you? More than that, it feels like it was meant for you? It takes you to a whole new understanding that you simply can't unlearn once you know it? This happened to me, around the time I was contemplating ending my relationship. The question I was asking was, should I stay here in safety and comfort, or leave and find safety in the future so I can say I've truly lived my life? I was tossing up the question, staring at my bookshelf, feeling bleak and lost, when an old book someone had recommended to me years earlier beckoned me to open it. The book was *The Tibetan Book of Living and Dying* by Sogyal Rinpoche. On my first attempt to read this tome I made it one quarter of the way through and had to put it down. I felt attacked by the piercing teachings. It's such an intensely truthful text that it slaps your ego, your understanding of yourself, right in the face. And my ego didn't like that very much. I hadn't been ready for the practice of detachment and rigid truth of Buddhism when I first picked up that book at age twenty-one. For years the book had been waiting for me to come back—and for some reason, on this particular day, I found the book again and opened it up to a random page. The page I opened outlined the exact message I needed to hear. It was what I had been seeking. It read:

Just as when waves lash at the shore, the rocks suffer no damage, but are sculpted and eroded into beautiful shapes, so our characters can be molded and our rough edges worn smooth by changes. Through weathering changes we can learn how to develop a gentle but unshakable composure.[1]

A peace washed over me as a vision popped into my mind. There was a future version of me that I'd dream about sometimes. I'd write about her. She was calm and grounded and just flowed through her life. Her heart poured out love effortlessly. Life worked for her, not against her. The earth quivered under confident footsteps, her soles connected to it with invisible roots. Her energy was warm and tropical, smelling of coconut and roses, and she'd just been swimming, hair dripping salt water. She was smiling, fresh, glowing, and deliciously free. She knew the truths of life, and somehow she was okay with them. She had developed an unshakable composure.

And so, knowing with clarity what I was seeking now, I went after it.

If I was going to find this new future version of me, I needed to go beyond just the physical, psychological, and biochemical model of understanding anxiety. That part is helpful, of course, but if I really wanted to find my unshakable composure, I knew I had to look inward as well and ask myself bigger questions. I had to listen to the deeper part of myself and connect with my true nature and the conscious observer within me that I had long neglected. And, soon enough, the essence of that future version of me fused into my present reality.

The Anxiety
Reset Method

Week One: Tuning In

Where Does Anxiety Come From?

In modern life, high-functioning anxiety is something we've been set up to experience. This is especially the case if we lack tools to avoid being controlled by the world around us, which so easily provokes stress. Reasons to feel anxious and overwhelmed are everywhere we look, woven into the fabric of our history, culture, systems, and family values. We live in an anxiogenic (anxiety-inducing) environment.

Our society values hard work and hustle culture. We feel guilty for taking time off to rest. More than ever do we feel the pressure to have the perfect life. There are so many everyday circumstances that can easily press the anxiety button, and most people don't realize that the level at which they impact you can be reduced. This is where resilience comes in, which we are working on building together through this book. You have a level of resilience within you that can be patched up, strengthened, and built upon—or worn down. Anyone with a low level of resilience will be more easily triggered by the pressures and experiences of modern life. You are not alone in this: many people you know have experienced or will experience anxiety at some point in their lives.

Too Much Work

For a start, consider the pressure placed upon us in our work lives. Working hours have extended far beyond the nine to five. More people than ever are expected to work overtime, answering emails at midnight and waking up early to check them again. The amount of work an employee takes on is increasingly more than a one-person job.

The forty-hour work week was developed in the 1940s, at a time when one person in a household would go to work and earn an income, with that as their sole focus. All other household tasks would typically be taken care of by a spouse. Now, we often find one person overloaded, taking on both professional and household demands. We create to-do lists we can never complete, asking the impossible of ourselves. Work bleeds into our private lives. Incomes have stagnated while the cost of living and house prices in the United States have risen. A single income is not enough to keep up, especially for those with children. The notion of living to work, rather than working to have freedom to live and enjoy our lives, has become normal.

Lack of Time

It feels as though there is never enough time. How often do you hear your friends and family say how busy they are—or complain of this yourself? How often do you find yourself wishing you had more time to complete the mountain of tasks before you? While it might feel like your days are becoming shorter and you're not being productive enough, there's something deeper going on. Many of us are experiencing a mismatch between our unrealistic expectations of how much we should be getting done and the hours in our day. There will never be enough time if we choose to see it that way. We'll go into this in more detail later, but for now know that continuing to live your life as a race against the clock is bound to create anxiety.

Trauma

Many of us have unprocessed, unacknowledged, buried trauma stuck in our nervous systems. Some traumatic experiences can be subtle, and you may not even realize they've had a lasting effect on you. Trauma is more than just sexual abuse, war, car accidents, and physical violence. It can result from more everyday experiences such as a lack of emotional support from a parent, a relationship breakup, a medical diagnosis, bullying in high school, or an intimidating boss. No doubt the entire world has experienced some degree of trauma after moving through the global pandemic. Trauma is a part of life, but most of us have no idea how to identify it or what to do with it. We may even end up accidentally passing it on to others as we bump up against one another in conflict. While it is within our power to understand our trauma and grow from it, much anxiety comes from beliefs we've created as a result of these unaddressed, ever-present painful experiences.

News Overload

We see crises impacting distant communities readily reported in the news. We feel powerless, as in many cases we can do nothing to directly help these situations. Every day we are presented a picture of a dangerous, unpredictable, and unsafe world. It often feels like it's just getting worse and humanity is doomed. Notice how I used the words "feels like." This perspective isn't necessarily true.

Community Cutoff

Even before the pandemic we had become more cut off from community than ever before, with much of our contact occurring via screens. Eye contact on public transport is frowned upon; it's much more appropriate to keep to yourself. Machines now replace human beings at supermarket checkouts. No longer are we connecting with people down the street with a smile and a wave hello. Getting to know our neighbors takes too much time and energy. Many of us are now shopping online, perfectly able to run our lives without even leaving the house. As a result, we feel more alone in our worries and less able to share our burdens with the reassuring support of a community.

Social Media

Social media and advertising prey on our insecurities to sell us things that promise to make us happier. We are overly exposed to fake representations of life, comparing ourselves to edited ideals of beauty, false eyelashes, and smoke-and-mirrors luxury lifestyles. Trolling and judgment are products of the toxic side of social media. We are driven more than ever to pursue material values, chasing the lie that the new car, phone, dress, body, or makeover will bring us happiness. This is bound to fuel an anxious mind.

Disconnection from Nature

We have lost our connection with nature. We ignore and condemn its inconvenient rhythms and cycles, blasting our heating and cooling systems, staying indoors when it's wet outside. We're oblivious to the seasonal nature of fresh produce. We spend more time indoors than ever, away from the dirt, sunlight, fresh oxygen, and green panoramas that were regularly available to our ancestors' brains. Our eyes are deprived of the calming benefits of greenery and Mother Nature's comforting nurture, and our anxious minds are feeling it.

The Resilience Shield

On top of all the pressures listed here you may have financial tension, relationship stressors, a full-time job of raising children or other care responsibilities, plus society's expectations and your ever-so-busy lifestyle to juggle. It's no wonder you feel anxious. It's no wonder you've formed beliefs that perpetuate your brain's anxiety and fear responses. Understand here that the way your brain is reacting is perfectly healthy given the kind of environment you're living in. The anxiety you feel is not a sign of your inherent weakness or shortcomings. You are surrounded by triggers. Some of us are more vulnerable to these triggers than others, but we all have the opportunity to build our Resilience Shield so we are less reactive and more connected with who we really are.

While you can usually only change some of your circumstances, you do have the power to change your internal experience of the world. You can reduce the impact of the outside world by turning inward, working on yourself, and building your resilience to what triggers you. You can learn to step out of the societal ideas and old belief systems that aren't serving you and into who you really are. You can become more connected to your own sense of security and truth. This is about learning to place yourself in the calm eye of the storm, instead of swirling around in the endless chaos of life around you.

The Resilience Shield is a very useful concept to allow you to find this sense of peace inside yourself. I've included a visual representation of each of the components that help you build resilience to those anxiety triggers, so you feel calmer and more grounded in yourself more of the time—and more readily able to respond rather than react to the challenges that come your way. These components include: being aware of your thoughts; creating meaningful connections; connecting to nature; prioritizing sleep, rest, and fun; committing to movement; using stimulants prudently; balancing hormones; optimizing gut health; and meeting your nutritional needs.

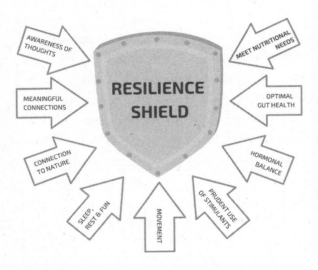

Whenever you feel the call of anxiety, come back to the Resilience Shield. Let it offer you some practical answers to explain why anxiety is asking for your attention. It can help you highlight the forgotten nurture points that you can then put some energy into and build upon. We will go through each component in detail in this book, spending the greatest amount of time working on thought awareness—as this is the one that requires the most attention and practice every single day.

While watching your mind and shifting it out of its fear stories is important, some days you feel so wound up that it is really hard to sit down and meditate, or even muster the strength to be aware of your thoughts. This is when it helps to have your physiology on your side. That means that you are meeting your nutritional requirements to create and release calming brain chemicals such as gamma-aminobutyric acid (GABA), serotonin, and dopamine. It means ensuring your gut health is optimal, so your gut bacteria can function at their best to send chemical signals along the vagus nerve to favorably shift the brain toward a calmer state. It means noticing and addressing your hormonal balance, lessening the impact of hormonal fluctuations that can increase anxiety and lower your mood. It means taking a good look at your use of stimulants such as caffeine, and prioritizing movement on most days. It means setting the appropriate time aside and adjusting conditions for a good night's sleep. It means making time for rest and fun, without pressure or guilt, and connecting back to nature, family, and friends.

When all the key components of the Resilience Shield are addressed, your whole body supports you in doing that inner work of exploring your limiting beliefs, questioning your fears, and processing negative emotions. Each component of the Resilience Shield will become much more familiar as we move through the Anxiety Reset Method.

Meet the Anxious Mind

Have you ever noticed that there is a voice inside your head narrating your entire life? It comments on how unattractive you look as you're brushing your teeth in the morning. It forecasts how your day will unfold, often with a negative filter. It starts planning what you're going to write in an email when you're in the middle of a yoga class. It even wants to prepare the next thing you're going to say to your friend when they're telling you a totally unrelated story. We tend to refer to this voice as the mind. Often the thoughts you think have no useful purpose for the moment you're in right now. These sentences running through your mind, like crimson news headlines on a television screen, are usually negatively skewed, unhelpful, and untrue. The thoughts and opinions of your mind are not the best source of information. To understand that you are not your thoughts is the most liberating gift you can give yourself. All of a sudden, you are free.

When anxiety was at its worst for me, I believed every word my mind told me. "You're not pretty enough. You're not working hard enough. They don't like you. You're never going to be happy. This thing you want isn't possible. You're so lazy. You'll probably do a terrible job. You look so stupid." On and on it went. Are you believing everything your mind tells you too? Do you *have* to believe your thoughts? What if the thoughts you're thinking are not actually true?

My mind still tempts me to believe my thoughts every day, but these days I soon become aware of what has happened and choose not to go with them. I learned that my mind would always tell particular stories and try to protect me with its fears and doubts. As I started to identify those stories, it became obvious to me how often they repeated—like broken records playing over and over—to the point where I started to see them as nothing new and rather uninteresting. "Oh, here's the story about how I am not good enough, again. Look at that, like clockwork I'm starting to doubt my abilities, just like I have done so many times before, and it always ends up being untrue. How boring." I learned to step outside all that noise and see that I was so much more. And so are you.

I wish we were taught how to effectively operate the machinery of our minds from the very beginning, way back in our early schooling. The mind can become your prison if you let it—if you never learn how to detach from it and access the truth. The mind can also be a loyal servant, helping you access more confidence, freedom, and new opportunities in your life, depending on what you tell it to think. Left unconscious, that mind will spit out all kinds of harmful ideas about you. I obediently believed what my mind told me—that I wasn't good enough or capable, that life was a struggle and bad things were going to happen to me. When I learned how to separate myself from my mind, everything changed. I suddenly found I could feel a sense of peace away from those thoughts whenever I needed to. Even better, I could start changing my thoughts to influence my emotional state. There are a few key things to understand if you want to do this too.

Think of your experience of your life as like looking through a pair of glasses. The glasses represent your mind's perspective as it thinks, judges, critiques, and solves problems. The glasses may be foggy, or covered in dust and someone else's fingerprints, or clouded with fear. When you realize you are wearing these glasses and take them off for a second, you can see with your true self—a self that feels and senses the truth beyond what the mind says. This is the pure, loving part of you. Other ways to describe the true self include your intuition, the observer, your heart, your higher self, your soul, or the witness. I may interchange between these terms from time to time, but for simplicity's sake they all mean your true self. In essence there is a fear-based-mind part of you, as well as a loving true-self part of you through which you can observe everything peacefully. The distinction between these two perspectives will become clearer as I explain more about the mind.

The mind is the thought-generating part of your brain that chatters away all day. It often imagines things going wrong. It criticizes you constantly. It's like living with your own worst enemy in your head. Know that feeling?

The mind is an expert at finding problems. This is what makes it important in some ways, because you do need your mind to help you function in life and stay alive. You can think of this as *useful thinking*. In prehistoric times we needed to understand how to collect wood, make a fire, and keep ourselves warm. We needed to know how to acquire food to nourish our bodies and fix a broken tool. If there was a saber-toothed tiger lurking around, we needed our minds to respond to the danger and ensure it was safe to go to sleep for the night. The mind is the reason we have evolved and survived so well over tens of thousands of years.

But nowadays we collect our food (often in its prepared state) from the supermarket, or order it to our door from our phones. We keep warm by pressing a button on the wall to switch on the heating. When it comes to our physical survival needs, most of them are readily met. We live so much more comfortably in the physical sense than our ancestors did.

However, the mind is still good at finding problems and "protecting" you. When it doesn't have many physical threats to work with, it needs a new target. So it starts focusing on *you*. It builds a strong case for why you are not good enough. It assesses whether or not people like you. It makes you question whether you are on the right path or really happy in your life. It takes guesses at all the future scenarios that could go wrong for you.

Then big life events happen. A divorce. Someone gets sick. You lose your job. When you are triggered by events in your life, you move into survival mode. The mind tries incessantly to find some kind of safety, certainty, and control. But for a lot of your problems, there is no satisfying solution to grasp on to right away. It doesn't matter how much analytical thinking and worrying you spin around in your head—there is often no answer that can soothe you in the short term. After a relationship breakup, for example, sometimes it just sucks for a while and there's nothing you can do to fix the problem, other than move through it and process the emotional pain. Many of the deep-rooted beliefs making you unhappy and anxious are hidden to you too. You probably aren't even aware of all the ways your parents and culture impacted you growing up, programming limiting, closed-off belief systems into you (albeit unconsciously).

Then there's the problem of endless problems. Solve one and another pops up, like a game of Whac-A-Mole. Life is full of problems if we allow the mind to constantly search for them. This is where useful thinking becomes unhelpful, ruminating, anxious thinking.

The mind is important and helpful, until it's not. Much of the time, the stream of endless thoughts from the mind is completely useless to you. You think a futile thought, such as "I'm not as good as them" or "I'm too shy" or "I'm so stupid," and you take that in as fact. You add that to your character profile, deciding that's who you are—even when it's not true. It is just a story you started telling yourself—an editable working file that you believe has been printed out and laminated. The story can be changed as you choose which thoughts to let in and which to let pass on by. You must understand that thoughts are just thoughts. They are not reality. They're ideas and mind junk, pouring out of your stream of consciousness. The mind generates thoughts that make you feel anxious and unsafe, yet most of these thoughts are dramatic, irrelevant, and not even the truth. Start seeing through them now. As you see through these self-harming thoughts, you can say to yourself, "Oh, look, that's fear. That's doubt. That's the mind. It's not me." You can remember to take off your mind's clouded glasses and see with your true self.

The first story to stop telling yourself is this: that you're an anxious person. It's time to stop using the labels the mind has attached to anxiety. Avoid referring to anxiety as something you possess—for example, calling it "*my* anxiety." You don't own that anxiety, just as you can't hold on to the thrill of delight you feel when you laugh at a joke. You are a person who experiences moments of anxiety, along with moments of many other emotions. Lean in to the spacious relief that comes with opening up to this idea. Who you are is so much more than your limited, fear-based mind would have you believe.

Mental Notes

- Your mind's thoughts and opinions are often not a trustworthy source of information.
- Your thoughts are not who you are. They are just thoughts.
- The mind can engage in useful thinking or unhelpful, anxious thinking.
- When you notice harmful, fear-based thoughts, you can bring awareness to them by saying to yourself, "That's the mind. It's not me."

Don't Hate Your Mind

When I teach this concept in my online program I notice many people begin to speak down to their mind. But to hate your mind is to fight against your humanness and your experience of life. That is not the direction we ideally want to move toward. I encourage you to laugh at your mind instead, like it's a child who doesn't know any better and is trying to do things like a grown-up. You might think of your mind like a puppy learning to walk on a leash, leaping onto a busy road with oncoming traffic. "Oh, look at my silly mind!" you might say to yourself, as you notice how it is fixating on what to cook for dinner when it's 9 a.m. and you're not even near a grocery store. Or perhaps your mind is imagining how stressful it will be giving that work presentation, bringing the pressure of that moment to life in your body right now—even though the actual event is a month away. "Isn't it interesting that my mind has come up with that?" you might say. Can you find it mildly amusing that the mind envisages all possible worst-case scenarios like that? Can you at least find it curious that the mind wants to put its focus there when it has no relevance to your life right now?

You can be grateful to your mind for the important work it does in solving logical life problems for you. You can also acknowledge that in almost every other endeavor, your mind—with its stream of thoughts that lures you away from the present moment—is essentially useless. Reducing the mind's importance is really helpful for putting its incessant thoughts down and finding more presence in your life. Of course, it's not always easy to do that when you feel anxious. That's because your relationship with your anxious thinking is all mixed up.

The Dog at the Door

Understanding the way anxiety works is the single most powerful thing you can do to outsmart it and, ultimately, master it. The trouble is, most of us respond to anxiety in a way that only feeds the fear and makes it worse.

When you experience anxiety, you may have noticed your instinct is to get rid of it as soon as possible. That's because your mind wants to move you away from pain and toward pleasure or pain relief. You want to run away from the discomfort fast, because it's really unpleasant to sit still when you're feeling anxious or stressed. You try to distract yourself or numb your senses—anything to just make it stop. You naturally speed up in your mind and live in the future, so you can plan ahead and predict what will happen next. That feels safer somehow. You imagine it will make you feel better if you can know what dangers might be coming for you. Or you overthink, trying to gain control that way. You believe that if you just think long and hard about the problem, you'll find the solution. Then you'll feel peaceful. Then you'll be able to fall asleep. After all the problems have been solved, it will be okay.

But, like a mirage of a luscious oasis in the desert, the peace on the other side keeps moving farther and farther away every time you try to get near it. You'll never find peace in this approach. What happens instead is that you feed the anxious mind more of what it wants: more problems, more distress, more energy and resistance. The anxiety only gets bigger.

It is completely normal to react to your anxiety this way. However, you must understand that these are all ineffective attempts at finding the kind of control you are after. When you notice yourself falling into these patterns, well done. Congratulate yourself. You have made progress with anxiety just by having that awareness. Now your mind can start understanding that this is not the best way to get out of the pain.

Let's look at this another way. Imagine you've left your pet dog outside in the rain. He's scratching at the door and barking, trying to get your attention so that you'll let him inside. You try yelling at him to stop, you try ignoring him, and you try thinking of new ways to get him to calm down. Maybe if you throw him a treat, he'll stop. The dog is distracted for a moment, but it doesn't take long before he is back at the door making lots of unpleasant noise. The longer you ignore him, the more distressed the dog becomes. The only way he's going to calm down is if you allow him to come inside the house to be with you. Maybe you need to give him some attention and towel him off so he's dry. Only then, inside the house, close and connected to you, will the dog be peaceful. It won't take long for him to fall asleep at your feet.

The dog in this story is your anxiety, and you've probably been managing it in a very ineffective way for a long time. There's one sure-fire way to find genuine control around anxiety, and it goes against all our instincts. I wonder if you've ever asked yourself this before: What if you allowed that anxious feeling to just be there? What if it was okay to feel the discomfort? What if you even welcomed it in, like letting the dog into your house?

Mental Notes

- When you fight the feeling of anxiety, you feed the fear and it gets worse.
- You have the ability to sit with the discomfort of anxiety.
- The most effective way to stop feeling anxious is to move toward that feeling and invite it in.

You Are the Blue Sky

It's normal to believe that the anxiety you feel is a part of you: a monster enveloping you and swallowing you whole. This is what happens when you lack awareness around what anxiety really is. As soon as you gain this new understanding, you move into a position of power over it quite quickly. You realize the anxiety is not who you are after all, but something separate from you.

The first step is recognizing that anxiety is just a sensation in your body. Yes, it is an intense feeling taking place in one part of you—maybe your chest or your gut—but it does not make up all of you. The uncomfortable sensation can't hurt you. It can only operate as a moving wave of intensity that will always change as the moments go by. The intensity level never stays the same for long. It will always pass. The overwhelm of emotion you feel comes from what you see in your imagination, the thoughts and stories your mind is telling you (whether conscious or unconscious), and the release of adrenaline and other stress hormones into your bloodstream. On the physical level, moment by moment, anxiety is not doing any real harm to your body. It's just causing an accelerated heartbeat, a heaviness in your chest, a churning sensation in your stomach, a restlessness in your limbs, a ball in your throat, and a short, shallow breathing pattern—or whatever sensations you usually experience.

The only way to truly move through an experience of anxiety is by learning to detach from it and see it for what it is. Just a sensation; an experience. Anxiety is not even a bad thing to feel, it's just that you've been labeling it as bad. It's simply a feeling that peaks with intensity and dies down after a few moments, like an ocean wave. Can you see anxiety as a neutral, interesting experience moving through your body?

Remember, the mind is only comfortable with the idea of moving you away from pain, toward relief. Once you practice this enough, your mind will learn that true relief lies on the other side of sitting with the sensation of anxiety. Choosing to label anxiety as neutral and avoiding words like "unbearable" or "attack" to describe it really helps your mind get on board with the whole idea. When you understand this, you realize that you are more than the anxiety—you can mentally sit back from it and see it from a distance. That is where you find control.

My clients often find that using an image of a blue sky is useful here. You, your true self, are the blue sky. The emotions you feel, including any negative emotions such as sadness, anger, disappointment, frustration, or anxiety, are just weather passing through. Perhaps there's a storm rolling in right now, representing the anxiety you feel. The blue sky exists at all times behind those storm clouds. Who you truly are, your true self, is still there underneath the blustering, whirring sensation in your gut, the spinning twister of thoughts in your mind. When you can simply let the anxiety move through your blue sky, knowing it is separate from you, you get a sense of detachment from it. You can see it from a distance, watching it pass by from a place of shelter, instead of being caught in the storm yourself. How powerful does this idea feel to you? This power is within you, and we're going to practice it. This is how you take control.

Mental Notes

- Anxiety is a neutral sensation moving through your body. It is neither good nor bad.
- Once you start observing the anxious feeling in this way, you see that you are separate from it, and you feel so much more in control.

How to Tune In

The words in this book can only guide you to your own experience of gaining mastery over your anxious mind. You have to implement the practices to experience what these words are trying to teach you. So, I invite you to try this little experiment: I call it tuning in. Read through the following instructions, then close your eyes and follow as much as you can remember in your head. Alternatively, you can hold the page open before you and peek at the words as you need guidance.

Start by closing your eyes. Take a deep breath into your belly, as you may have done in a meditation before. Take as many slow, deep breaths as you need to settle into a calmer state. Be mindful of the shifting of your clothes as you breathe in, the way your chest expands, the feeling of the air moving through your nostrils and fresh oxygen flooding into your bloodstream. Feeling more settled, eyes closed, you're ready to focus on the black screen before you.

At first the mind will be very active, reminding you to remember what you need to do later or bringing up that big problem you have that still needs solving. Notice that urge within you, pulling you back into thought: "Maybe if I just keep thinking about it, I'll find the solution." Remind yourself that this is anxious, unhelpful thinking. It doesn't get you the control you want. Just feel into the understanding that it is okay to set that thinking aside for now, to put it down, to allow it to be less important. The thoughts don't have to stop completely. They never will. Zero thinking is not the aim here. The only thing to aim for is a greater awareness of those thoughts, like you're rising up out of them and looking at them from a distance. What exactly are the sentences moving across the black screen, like news-ticker headlines at the bottom of a TV broadcast? What story is your mind running right now? If you had to write down a thought sentence or two, what words would you put on paper? Can you really try to see your thoughts as words?

It doesn't matter what the thoughts are, how mundane or useless they seem. All you're doing now is practicing noticing the thoughts. During this process you'll lose your focus and forget, and get lost within a thought once more. That's normal. When you eventually realize you have lost focus, gently and with self-kindness draw your awareness back to the thoughts. Watch them like fallen leaves floating on the surface of a river. Let them drift on by.

You are thinking thoughts all day, every day. The vast majority of your thoughts slip past your awareness entirely. They can be so hidden from your conscious awareness that you don't even realize that your thoughts are just sentences: collections of random words and images in the mind.

As you get more comfortable with the concept of watching the thoughts, start to imagine you are a hawk, alert and focused. You're flying above an open landscape, eyeing it for movement, waiting for a mouse to appear. Enjoy the focused attention, the resting of your awareness on that central place you've found in the black screen. The mouse represents your next thought. As you wait for the mouse to appear, you can experience another part of yourself. Can you notice that emptiness between each thought? Even for a moment, in the waiting for the next thought, there is space. There is a brief pause, a moment of nothing, of stillness, just before the next thought arrives. Just sit with the feeling of being connected to a *you* that is not caught in your mind's stream of thoughts, even if it only lasts for one second. In that one second, the weight of the world, of caring what people think and needing to be responsible or do something productive to prove your worth, lifts. Life is light. There is relief, peace, and presence. It's like taking a holiday from your busy mind.

If you can do this, you have experienced an awareness of the two parts of yourself we discussed earlier. If there is a mind part of you that thinks and another presence within you that sees the thinking mind, who is this presence watching the mind? There is the mind that thinks thoughts, and there is the part of you that is observing the thoughts as they move across the mind. This part of you is what I have referred to as the loving true self.

Now scan your body and notice any sensation of anxiety or any kind of negative emotion. Be with the sensation as it moves through you, watching it with curiosity and without judgment. Can you allow the anxiety you feel to simply be a sensation, neither good nor bad? Can you keep your hawk-like focus locked onto the sensation? Can you allow yourself to soften around the anxious feeling as you continue to observe it with pure awareness? Can you feel the relief as the feeling weakens and releases all by itself, without you having to do anything other than watch it?

If you've connected to this concept and have experienced for a moment what it is to embody the higher-self version of you, the true self that rises above the thinking mind, you have succeeded in this first important step toward successfully and profoundly mastering your anxious mind.

Soon enough you'll begin to relate to any moment of anxiety with this powerful tool, giving you a compelling feeling that you can withstand the discomfort whenever you feel it. Just knowing that you have this ability will mean you fear the anxiety less, and anxiety will start to visit you far less frequently, with less intensity than ever before.

Practice

This week, practice tuning in to the experience of anxiety. I suggest spending two minutes doing this upon waking, sometime during the day such as before a meal, and just before bed. It need only take a minute or so of focused awareness with your eyes closed, like a mini meditation. If you haven't quite experienced the release of anxiety yet, keep practicing. It will come the more you enter the process from the calm confidence of your true self, watching the sensation like you're shining a torch of awareness upon it, giving it all your attention, without judging it as bad or trying to change it.

Changing Your Beliefs

As you learn these new concepts, read over these words, challenge your thinking, and apply these practices, you are actively dismantling and rebuilding your belief systems. Changing your beliefs is a crucial factor in creating transformation in your life and mastering anxiety.

While it would be great to separate from your thoughts all day long, this isn't realistic for most people. The mind will always be there, thinking thoughts. You can't switch it off, no matter how much you meditate. Instead, you can empower yourself by starting to influence some of those thoughts and the way they make you feel. You can start to choose the habits of thought your mind cycles around.

Remember that thoughts are random mind junk, usually irrelevant to the moment you're in now and not necessarily true. The beliefs you hold are the thoughts that you think over and over. Every day you wake up and think pretty much the same thoughts. You look in the mirror and the same thoughts about your appearance arise. You have to be in a hurry, because your thoughts tell you that the race of life is on again. You reflect on your schedule and you think about how you are dreading the day ahead. These thoughts become entrenched in your mind as beliefs. You start to believe your life is as bleak, joyless, and frightening as your thought patterns make out.

But a thought is literally just a thought. It's a nonphysical idea floating somewhere in your mind. A thought like "I'm such a bad person" holds as much weight as a thought like "I wonder what pink elephants eat for breakfast?" And as you know by now, the mind isn't a great source of trustworthy, self-serving information.

There will always be negative, unhelpful thoughts in your mind that you wouldn't choose to be there. While you can't choose every thought, it doesn't mean you have *no* power here. You can actively choose *some* thoughts. In fact, by choosing thoughts actively each day, you can exert a great deal of power over your emotional well-being and how you respond to the world.

Every time your brain receives a new thought that you've never had before, your brain cells form new networks. This process occurs within milliseconds. It is impossible to be aware of this process as it happens too quickly. Each brain cell can form thousands of networks in response to new information.

At first, these networks are not very strong. They are more like a single electrical wire, as opposed to a thickened electrical cable made of bundles of wires wound together. A new thought first forms as one of these weaker single wires. It's unfamiliar to the mind and might feel strange. Over time, though, as you deliberately and consistently practice the new way of thinking, the wire gets stronger and bundles together with other wires to form a thick cable. This cable is strong and won't be removed.

Consider how strong the electrical cables in your brain might be regarding fear, anxiety, and negative thought patterns. Right now, as we're only just beginning this work, your old cables are really tough. When you deliberately prioritize new ways of thinking, your old networks can be trimmed back within a matter of days, or even hours. It takes time to form new habits. I always instruct my clients to listen to their hypnotherapy audio tracks for at least twenty-one days. In that amount of time, you stop using those old pathways and start using new ones. The wires connecting to the old way of being literally fall away with lack of use. How exciting it is to think these old beliefs don't have to come back unless you deliberately choose them again. This is why the work of changing your beliefs is so transformational and long-lasting, and so worth the effort of applying the practices in this book.

What if you focused upon and built your preferred brain connections daily? What if you started feeding your mind thoughts that you already *are* the calm, confident, more present, and relaxed person you want to be? What if you started believing you are already a whole new version of yourself?

This is how you change your beliefs and reset your anxious mind. You stop thinking the old thoughts as often by becoming more conscious of them. You start thinking new thoughts and spending more time immersed in them. You don't have to do it perfectly. You don't have to think new thoughts all day, every day. However, if you open your mind to the new thoughts and let yourself believe them for ten seconds more today than yesterday, you are starting to change your brain. If you spend ten seconds less thinking the unhelpful, limiting thoughts, you are going to start to change. It's all about building those new networks in your brain. As you spend your time reading through this book, you are actively taking in new thoughts and new information, building new connections in your brain, and creating a whole new version of yourself in the process.

The most important belief you must begin to shift is the belief that you are an anxious person—like it's a personality trait, your identity, or an intrinsic part of you. Notice I've mentioned this several times already. This is deliberate, because each time it runs through your mind, the thought becomes more and more familiar to you. Anxiety is an experience you have in life sometimes. It's a sensation in your body that you are used to feeling. It's tied up in thoughts that you are used to thinking. Anxiety is a habit you have developed, but it is not who you are. And we are breaking that circuit.

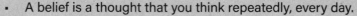

Mental Notes

- A belief is a thought that you think repeatedly, every day.
- Beliefs change when you become conscious of and stop thinking old thoughts, and when you actively choose to think new thoughts.

The Power of Movement

While tuning in is a foundational tool I encourage you to use regularly, there are other ways to reduce your susceptibility to feeling triggered into anxiety in the first place. There is a tool to reduce anxiety that is completely free of charge, that anyone can access, without nasty side effects. It can help you feel even stronger and more in control. Does this sound too good to be true?

Movement is the first physical component we will address in building your anxiety resilience. The physiological components of this work are just as important as the mental concepts we've been exploring so far. This one is so important that it needs to come first—before the gut healing, the hormone balancing, and the nutrition.

Remember your pet dog we talked about earlier? What would happen if you skipped a few days of taking him for a walk? Imagine you don't have a big backyard for him to explore. A daily walk is his one opportunity to expend a lot of energy, but he is denied this chance. He's kept inside. How would your dog respond? Would he be calm and relaxed, sleeping on the floor all day? Or would he be restless, fidgety, and even destructive, chewing up your new pair of shoes? And doesn't that sound a lot like anxiety?

Remember that you are an animal too. If you don't go for walks or move your body in some way, you will likely feel more anxious. Consider for a moment how anxiety often feels like an urge to move, like you need to get going. When you do move regularly, you are giving yourself the movement your body craves. You have stored-up energy that needs to be used in a healthy way each day—and not just from overthinking.

In one significant study, researchers evaluated the impact of exercise on anxiety symptoms. They combined the results of forty-nine different trials, gathering evidence from 3,500 people, and found that exercise alone is effective in managing anxiety.[1] Nothing else is required. This means that for many people with anxiety, medication and conventional psychotherapy are not necessarily needed to feel better. Movement is that powerful.

Next, the researchers wanted to know how people experienced anxiety when using exercise as a stand-alone therapy compared to those receiving support through conventional psychotherapy and medication. Interestingly, they found that exercise is just as effective as psychotherapy and medication for managing anxiety. The results in each group were more or less the same. It blows my mind that this information isn't more widely discussed. Rarely do we hear exercise talked about as the first go-to therapy for anxiety—certainly not compared to traditional talk therapy and medication prescriptions. More recently, another group of researchers suggested that doctors should be encouraging exercise as a frontline treatment for anxiety, given that it is so safe and effective.[2]

Making decisions and taking action can be challenging when you are experiencing anxiety. Exercise improves cognition, increases blood flow to the brain, and even grows the prefrontal cortex—the decision-making part of the brain that helps us to set goals, work toward them, and take action. Exercise also increases our brain-derived neurotrophic factor (BDNF). BDNF is like the brain's cushion for stress, protecting it from damage. It supports brain cell survival, growth, and function. Healthy brain cells facilitate calmer, clearer thinking. When you have higher levels of BDNF, the brain's fear activation response is lower. You're less likely to react with anxiety to a stressful trigger. Those who exercise also tend to recover better from post-traumatic stress disorder and recurring panic attacks.[3] A well-functioning, healthy brain supports your anxiety resilience.

So what type of exercise is most effective for anxiety? Aerobic-style movement can be beneficial, such as brisk walking, swimming, running, dancing, bike riding, and high-intensity interval training (HIIT). However, any movement that increases your breathing and heart rate is good. The most important thing is to make sure you enjoy the movement you choose. This is for you and your state of mind. Whether you love the idea of walking, surfing, hiking in nature, or kickboxing, choose an activity you can see yourself sticking to and make it your sacred practice to commit to. If you've always been interested in Pilates, yoga, or martial arts, get curious about how fun it could be to explore those activities. Maybe you could join a gym or seek a personal trainer to give you some guidance.

Aim to do some kind of movement every day, even if it's a fifteen-minute walk or five minutes of dancing in your bedroom. You know your body, your fitness level, and your ability, and you can work out what will suit you best. I encourage you to tune in to your body and do what feels good. Overexercising and pushing yourself to exhaustion can increase the body's stress load. If you're already very active and exercising daily, check in with yourself. You might need to pull back a little and allow one to two rest days.

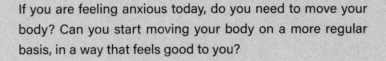

Practice

If you are feeling anxious today, do you need to move your body? Can you start moving your body on a more regular basis, in a way that feels good to you?

Week One Checklist

For this first week, you have two practices to work on. Revisit the sections How to Tune In and The Power of Movement for more detailed explanations.

☐ Practice tuning in for two minutes, three times per day. Notice how the way you relate to moments of anxiety changes with this powerful tool.

☐ Set an intention to move your body regularly to shift anxious energy. If you're feeling anxious, consider how much you have moved that day.

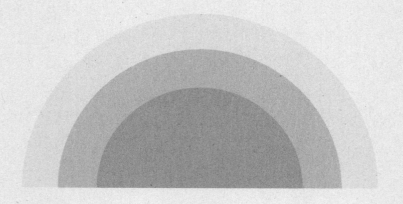

Week Two: Understanding Anxiety

Anxiety Has a Message

Now that you understand the basics of the anxious mind, you might be wondering why the uncomfortable sensation of anxiety pops up so often. Is there some kind of point to the storm clouds that mess up our beautiful blue skies? Just as we need the rain to nourish the land, we need anxiety and fear to push us where we need to go: to grab our attention, to keep us in balance, to put us back on track.

Your anxiety is calling out to you, whether you like it or not. It always has something to say—it's just that most of us don't listen because it's so damn uncomfortable and we just want it gone. We hate it. We push it away. We deny it its voice.

I'm with you in acknowledging that this part of anxiety sucks. Let's not pretend it is fun. But you *can* build a healthier relationship with the anxiety you feel by appreciating that there's something very useful and true hidden within it. If you're going to master your anxious mind, you need to grasp the value in it.

Have you ever taken a moment to ask the anxiety why it is here? What if you listened to what it is trying to tell you? Is there an issue you need to address? Is there something inauthentic about the way you're living your life, your career, or your relationships that is setting off that warning signal?

Our bodies are wired with an alarm system to tell us when our fundamental needs are not being met. When we feel anxious, it is always for a reason. The reason may be spiritual, psychological, or physical. The Resilience Shield I introduced in Week One may already have given you some significant clues. Understanding and running through your basic mental health needs (we'll talk about those later in this chapter) will also provide insights. Regardless, the message in the anxiety is something to welcome and try to understand.

Sometimes you feel anxious simply because your body needs more sleep, or because you're not eating regular meals and your blood sugar levels are unstable. Sometimes there is anxiety because you're in a situation that isn't serving you. Maybe you're hanging around certain people who aren't very kind to you, or you're ignoring the call to follow a big, scary dream that will help you grow. Instead of reverting to the easy answer—that anxiety happens for no reason—let's dig a little deeper. Believing that anxiety is meaningless can leave you feeling helpless, instead of encouraged to take back your power and learn how to harvest anxiety's gifts.

Practice

What are the most common messages your anxiety brings you? Can you take a few guesses? If you don't know, get curious and ask yourself what you'd write down if you *did* know.

For example, the anxiety might be saying you need to take better care of yourself, learn to be kinder to yourself, leave a toxic workplace, cultivate friendships that align with your true self, or follow your heart's calling.

Don't worry about getting this perfect right now. You'll have a chance to develop these ideas as we continue.

When You Ignore the Message

You've no doubt been stuck in the anxiety loop for a long time. It can feel like sitting on a merry-go-round of thoughts you can't seem to get off. Now, as you have started tuning in and noticing you can find a few moments of stillness off that merry-go-round, you may be wondering why you have been stuck in this cycle for so long. As you now understand, your thoughts are not who you are; when you lack this awareness and you're caught up in the storm of anxious thinking, it feels uncomfortable and sometimes painful—and you just want a break. You want it to stop.

In seeking a quick way out of the anxiety, you end up missing the message. The dog at the door barks louder, but you manage to quiet it down a little with your coping mechanisms. For some of us, this looks like food and emotional eating. For others, it's shopping, endlessly scrolling on social media, smoking, drinking alcohol, gambling, working longer hours than necessary, taking drugs, watching too much porn, having a lot of risky sex, or getting lost in the highs (and lows) of a romantic relationship or string of relationships. Your coping mechanisms may well include several of these—anything that will give you a little hit of distraction or dopamine, or numb the pain. It is worth clarifying that many of these activities are not inherently bad, it just depends on the context in which you engage in them. Are you using them only to distract yourself from having to be present with uncomfortable feelings? Or are they genuine celebrations and pleasures in your life? There can be healthier ways to distract yourself too, such as exercise, but most unhealthy coping mechanisms have a detrimental effect on you—and sometimes those around you—over time.

These coping mechanisms are your attempts to find peace, to feel connected to something, to feel loved and content for a few moments when you don't have any better tools available to you. Engaging in them is your own way of regulating your nervous system.

Everyone has their coping mechanisms. There is nothing to be ashamed of, because all of us are innately driven to connect. If you are feeling disconnected from yourself, as so many of us do, you will develop these tendencies. When you don't want to feel the uncomfortable sensations of negative emotions in your body, you are disconnecting from feeling. You are pretending that you are not sensitive, exhausted, sad, disappointed, or scared. You are hiding away from your true feelings. You're disconnecting from yourself.

Food in particular is ingrained in us as the quickest way to feel better from a very young age—like when a crying child is given a lollipop. Emotional eating is one of the most common coping mechanisms I see in people with high-functioning anxiety. The anxiety you feel is a yearning to connect back to yourself, a warning signal that you aren't connected to your true self. Of course, the food only numbs the feeling for a moment. The kind of connection the anxiety is calling you to is deeper than that, and one that only you can give to yourself. We will explore this in more detail soon.

To figure out why you've been stuck in the anxiety cycle for so long, you must first consider this: How long have you been ignoring the message to reconnect with yourself?

Practice

What do you do to cope, numb, or distract yourself from anxiety? Write down some ideas in your journal to bring more awareness to the coping mechanisms you've been leaning on. Remember that this is not an invitation to berate yourself with judgment. It is an opportunity to learn about your unconscious habits. From that place, with compassion for yourself, you will grow in your ability to choose differently (more of the time).

Meeting Your Basic Mental Health Needs

Each of us has a barometer of mental health that can go up and down, depending on how well we are meeting what I call our basic mental health needs. Whenever a client of mine is struggling to find the message in their anxiety, reviewing the basic mental health needs can be a really useful way to quickly find answers and see how to make helpful changes.

These needs are:

- Belonging and connection
- Certainty, control, and safety
- Choice and freedom
- Contribution and purpose
- Growth and learning
- Self-worth and significance

When you understand what these needs are, you can see which are lacking for you. We'll look at each of these needs in detail now. Come back to this section whenever you feel unsure of what the anxiety is trying to tell you. Armed with this knowledge, you can form your game plan and take action steps toward better meeting each need and improving your mental health on those days when you feel anxiety calling out for your attention.

Connection and Belonging

Why does it hurt so much when someone leaves us? Why is bullying so damaging? Why does rejection sting so badly? Why is it that social situations can be so nerve-racking?

Feeling connected to a group is a mental health need we all have. It goes deep into our survival instincts. Back in prehistoric times, if you were alone in the wilderness your chances of survival were pretty low. If you were part of a group of humans working together in a tribe, in contrast, there was someone to help you gather food, someone to care for you if you were sick or injured, and other minds to collaborate with to solve the day-to-day challenge of staying alive. That's why belonging to a group sends a message to your brain that you are safe and you are going to survive. When you are bullied, rejected, broken up with, abandoned, isolated, or left out, something in your brain says you are not going to be able to keep living. You're no longer safe. It feels like life or death to the mind.

We can achieve a sense of connection through maintaining healthy social relationships as well as a connection with ourselves on a spiritual level. As you connect with your true self, you can learn to trust that the connection is always there within you when you need it. This isn't to say you must become fully self-reliant and ignore relationships with others, but if you are relying on others to help you feel connected to a point where you have lost all of your power, you might want to work on strengthening that connection with yourself. You give your power away to others when you can't bear a week away from your partner, for example, because you're afraid you won't have your need for connection met during that time. You have the power to feel this connection within yourself, at all times. You also have a responsibility to satisfy your survival brain and enjoy the company of other people too. There is a balance.

So how can we meet our need for connection? The answer can vary from day to day, but you must make building a connection with yourself a priority. You may connect with yourself through a regular journaling practice, working with tuning in and sitting with your emotions, and allowing yourself the space to feel. You may also need to actively become more involved with a community of people and reach out to friends instead of waiting for someone to call you.

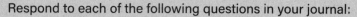

Practice

Respond to each of the following questions in your journal:
- How connected do you feel to yourself?
- Do you have an inner circle you can rely on for support?
- Do you feel like you belong?
- How could you feel more connected in your life?

Certainty, Safety, and Control

Why are we constantly planning for the future? Why do we so often turn to obsessive food or exercise regimes when life feels out of control? Why do we stay in our comfort zones? Why do we feel so anxious when we venture away from our tight schedules and routines?

If you're someone who knows high-functioning anxiety, it's probably no surprise that having a sense of control, safety, and certainty is a key mental health need. We like to know it's all going to work out okay. We want to see what's around the corner so we can make plans for it and be prepared. We want reassurance that our survival is no longer threatened. When our sense of certainty and safety is damaged, anxiety is bound to show up. This is exactly what happened to me when my parents split up and, as I described earlier, that sense of something solid and reliable in my life suddenly turned to sinking quicksand.

Safety is best found as a feeling you nurture within you rather than a circumstance outside you. If you can change a circumstance to feel safer, of course you can take action to make that happen. But so often the circumstances outside us are changing and out of our control.

Later in this process we will look at practices that build your sense of safety, so you can loosen your grip on control. For now, just start to consider some changes you could easily bring about to create more safety in your life—especially if there are obvious circumstances you've been ignoring that you can change. For example, it might not feel the safest right now to be going into a toxic workplace. Reaching out for support, making a plan to improve the situation, and talking to someone who can help could be ways to increase your sense of safety.

Practice

Respond to each of the following questions in your journal:
- How safe do you feel in your life?
- How certain do you feel that things will work out for you?
- What is it that you need to increase your sense of safety?
- How you could feel safer and more in control in your life?

Growth and Learning

We are part of an expanding universe. There is nothing more natural than growing and moving forward. It's no wonder that we crave it in our lives, and that our mental health suffers when we don't feel like we are making progress. Embrace the idea that expansion is your natural state. Progress feels good. If you aren't growing and learning, you feel stuck and stagnant. This can present as anxious restlessness. It's like you have unused energy and potential with nowhere to go.

Growth and learning might look like reading a new book, exploring a new topic that fascinates you, or following your curiosity. It might be taking up a new hobby, practicing a skill, or trying something different. It could be opening yourself up to the other side of an argument or an issue you care about, or learning about a different culture or perspective.

By choosing to read this book and work on your anxiety, you're already meeting this need to some extent. Where else could you keep growing? Consider your work, social life and relationships, spiritual journey, health, and personal development.

Practice

Respond to each of the following questions in your journal:
- Do you feel like you are growing and learning in all aspects of your life?
- How can you grow or learn more in the areas that need it?
- What is holding you back from expansion and growth?

Self-Worth and Significance

We all want to feel special. While we want to be part of the crowd and fit in, we also have a contrasting need: to feel different and unique. We want to stand out and be acknowledged for the greatness within us.

The ego does need to be kept in check here. Meeting the need for self-worth and significance is not about posting lots of selfies or focusing on your outward appearance. It's not about showing off your possessions and how much money you have, or trying to impress others. As we'll later discuss, this approach is not sustainable: It doesn't satiate your deeper sense of self-worth. The thrill of the compliment from a stranger or friend is short-lived, leaving you empty and hungry for more. External validation is an addictive cycle you need to be mindful of if you are to build deep self-worth, in which you validate and praise yourself.

Meeting this need in a healthy way requires you to learn to connect to the observing part of yourself: that part that watches your thoughts passing through the mind and sees the stories it tells. This true-self part of you is always enough, on time, loved, peaceful, and safe. There is greatness within this part of you, but the important bit is understanding that the greatness in you is also in others. Yes, you are inherently special and significant, but this does not need to come from a sense of superiority above others.

Practice

Respond to each of the following questions in your journal:

- How significant and worthy do you feel?
- Do you like yourself? Do you love yourself?
- What is it that you do or don't like about yourself? What parts of yourself are unacceptable to you? (Simply bring some awareness to this and leave it for now. We will work on this in more depth later.)

Choice and Freedom

While the anxious thinking will have you clinging to certainty and safe predictability at all costs, there's another need that contradicts this: the need for choice and freedom. The play between these two needs can make you feel incredibly confused and restless. We crave freedom, multiple choices, and, to some degree, a little uncertainty—a sense of surprise and adventure in our lives. Have you ever been in a romantic relationship and noticed how much you appreciate the security and safety someone provides but then also feel like it's a bit boring? That there's not enough adventure? This is a very common thought process to have regarding a relationship. We want someone who feels like home and an adventure all at once. It is important to note that you have this need, without letting it destroy all your relationships.

This need can apply to many aspects of our lives. You might have noticed yourself thinking your career or work just isn't exciting enough, even though it provides a secure income. And no, you're not asking for too much to want excitement in your life. But there are destructive ways to meet this need, such as jumping from one relationship to the next or constantly changing careers. There are healthier approaches to meeting this need.

I like to use the example of playing a computer game and knowing all the cheat codes. How quickly does the game become boring when you have complete control over it, knowing that you're going to win? Do you care as much when you remove the element of surprise in how it unfolds? Or imagine rewatching a movie you've already seen five times. It's just not the same when you watch it again, knowing that everything works out fine in the end. The same perspective can be applied to our lives. Are you beginning to see the appeal of some uncertainty in life? Not knowing how it's all going to go is a huge gift. Without it, we wouldn't ever experience the amazing feeling of awe and wonder.

For now, it is enough to understand that we like knowing there are surprises in store. We like having options to choose from. Just consider having no options in your life, and you'll feel it. We feel alive when we open up to possibilities and opportunities. We like having adventures, taking the road less traveled, choosing which way to go at the fork in the road, and exploring the world.

Practice

Respond to each of the following questions in your journal:

- Do you believe that you have choice and freedom in your life?
- Do you feel that there are opportunities waiting to be discovered?
- Could there be some wonderful surprises in store?
- Where could you create more freedom, choice, and that sense of inviting in the unexpected surprises in your life?

Purpose and Contribution

We like to move around in the world with purpose and meaning. We need a reason to get up in the morning, for being here on this planet. We like to know that our actions are valuable. We want to make a difference.

It is very normal to spend periods of your life seeking a purpose or a way to contribute. It's important that you don't judge yourself for feeling that you're lacking in this area. Many, many people also grapple with this in their lives. However, this doesn't mean that it isn't possible to create a deeply fulfilling life for yourself, no matter your circumstances. There is no perfect formula to finding your purpose, other than giving yourself permission to ponder your dreams, learning to connect with your inner wisdom, and breaking through limiting beliefs about what is possible. We will be exploring each of these concepts in detail throughout this book.

You get to decide the meaning of your life. This is a very powerful notion to become aware of. Most of us automatically choose ideas about how meaningful our life is from what others around us tell us. We seek their approval and validation. "Ah, you have a statue erected in your name, or millions of dollars, or you are famous. Now you have contributed to the world," a part of us waits to hear.

The meaning you choose will create the evidence you find in your life to back it up. So, if I decide my meaning is to help people, I'll automatically look for instances where helping people is showing up in my life, selecting more evidence to support this belief. If I decide my life has no meaning, the circumstances of life around me will naturally reveal a purposelessness to life. Life reflects the beliefs in your own mind. This is quite possibly the most powerful piece of information you can learn about life and taking back control of it. You have so much more power than you realize.

Practice

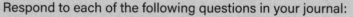

Respond to each of the following questions in your journal:

- Do you believe that your life has purpose?
- Do you feel that you are making a contribution to the world that is also fulfilling to you?
- What might your purpose be? What are your dreams and passions? (Don't worry if you're either coming up blank or you have some crazy ideas that you'd never tell anyone. This is just for you. There is time to come back to this question and explore it later in this book.)

Being Kind to Yourself

The mind—that voice that narrates your life—is usually oriented toward finding all the things that are wrong with you. It collects more and more evidence to prove its case that you are not enough as you are. This is the inner critic. I have one and you have one.

It's that voice that says "I look like shit today" or "What an idiot, why did I say that?" It's the unfriendly seeker of flaws. It keeps a record of every piece of negative feedback you've ever received in your life and tells you that it's probably true.

Sometimes it's more subtle, just nudging you with a poke of its finger that you should be more productive right now, or you really should have gone to the gym, even though you're exhausted. It keeps you striving for perfection, holds you to the highest standards, and shames you for falling short every time. "Of course you fell short," the inner critic says, "because there's something terribly wrong with you." Whenever you find yourself swimming in the sea of all that could be wrong with you—not smart enough, not pretty enough, not thin enough, not likable enough, not witty enough, not productive enough, not successful enough, not popular enough, and downright just not good enough in general—you know your inner critic is in full swing.

If you haven't spent much time bringing awareness to your inner critic, now is a great time to start noticing it. Give it a name, like Sheryl or Mona. Have you ever noticed that the voice of your inner critic actually sounds a lot like someone you know? It might be your mother, your father, a sibling, a schoolteacher, a grandparent, or anyone who had an influence on you growing up. You could even label your inner critic with their name, helping you sense a distance between you and this part of your mind.

The thing is, in its own weird way, the inner critic is trying to help you—just like the mind is trying to help you solve problems.

The inner critic wants to control what other people think of you. The logic goes something like this: "If I can identify and fix all my flaws first, before anyone else sees them, no one will find them and reject me for them." To the inner critic, rejection is the worst possible thing that could happen. Rejection is painful. It means being an outcast, being lonely, being left for dead, and not having that ever-so-vital need for connection and belonging met. We all know the feeling.

The irony is that you end up rejecting yourself, disconnecting from your own heart, and isolating yourself from the limitless source of love within you. And the craziest part of all is that *you* are the one person you most need acceptance from. You need your own approval far more than you need anyone else's.

The inner critic is based in fear. It's afraid that you are not enough as you are. It's the scared little child part of you, needing love, comfort, and support. And if indeed you've realized your inner critic does sound like a parent or caregiver, understand that the criticism you received from them came from their own scared little child too.

While the inner critic will always be there to some extent, you can learn to quiet its voice and reconnect with your inner kindness, which I call the loving parent within you. Becoming kinder to yourself is not something that comes naturally to most people. You must learn it like you've just decided to take up golf. It's a lifelong skill. You need patience and practice. At first it will feel strange as you swing your arms holding this new piece of equipment in a new way. You need to learn the steps, and you'll have to hit the ball several times and lose a few in a duck pond before you master it. It won't happen overnight, and it won't feel comfortable. Don't expect to be good at it or consistent with it right away. You may feel like you're fumbling or faking it and not doing it right, or it might feel silly. I've had clients who couldn't even say the words "I love you" to themselves without cringing or whispering it. However, when it came to telling me about everything that was wrong with them, their monologue was effortless.

It comes back to what is familiar to the mind. Right now, criticism is familiar to your mind. It has been conditioned that way, over years and years of repeating the same habitual thoughts. You learned to criticize yourself. You learned to doubt yourself. That's a great thing to recognize, because if you've already learned how to speak unkindly to yourself, that means you can learn how to speak to yourself with kindness, too.

Understanding perception is the key to unlocking the kind, loving voice within you. The way you perceive yourself is completely up to you. You might enjoy eating chocolate, but it's not the chocolate itself that is creating the pleasurable experience. It's your thoughts about how delicious and pleasant eating chocolate can be. Some people love chocolate and others hate it. I personally don't understand how anyone can hate chocolate, but it's true. Chocolate is not inherently good and delicious. It's the way you perceive it. This is why I can use hypnotherapy to train people to be disgusted by foods they feel addicted to, or why some people who have experienced a really bad hangover after consuming a specific type of alcohol find they cannot drink it ever again. The mind tells the story: "This is the poison that made me sick."

As such, no person and no object in this world is inherently beautiful. Growing up, I idolized Angelina Jolie as the most beautiful woman in existence, yet my brother disagreed. Her beauty wasn't the kind of beauty he liked. Art critics debate about the meaning of art and the genius of artists all the time. We've all looked at an acclaimed piece of art and thought, "Really? All that money and attention for *this*? A five-year-old could have made that." Each of us has unique preferences, likes and dislikes, past experiences, and social conditioning that skews our perception. You will even have a different perception depending on your mood, moment to moment. Perception is ever-changing and completely subjective. In other words, the value, worth, and enjoyment of anything in your life is for you to decide. Including everything about yourself.

So if you are free to choose your perception of you, why wouldn't you choose a positive one? Why wouldn't you tell yourself a story about you that serves you and encourages you to go after your dreams, making your life much more enjoyable?

You could take any human being on the planet and say they're not attractive enough, too old, boring, not smart enough, or too big. Equally, you could take any human being and say they're wonderful, interesting, strong, and intelligent. You could say they have a lovely smile, a big heart, and a beautiful soul. It's your choice to see yourself with criticism and let Sheryl or your mother's voice take over, or to talk to yourself like a best friend and build yourself up.

Researchers from the University of Melbourne found that women transitioning through menopause had a much lower likelihood of experiencing anxiety when they scored high on a self-compassion test.[1] Self-compassion is essentially letting yourself off the hook and being kind to yourself. It provides a protective effect. Becoming aware of your thoughts and the way you speak to yourself is also a key component of the Resilience Shield.

There has to come a time in your life when you just start practicing self-compassion, when you give it a try, even if it makes you cringe or feels fake, and you keep trying. You're here, working your way through this book. That time might as well be now.

Mental Notes

- The way you perceive yourself is completely up to you. No one else can choose it for you.
- Why wouldn't you actively choose a perception of yourself that builds your self-esteem?

Practice

Write a two-page self-love letter, answering the question: How am I lovable, perfect, and enough as I am? Consider your achievements, the elements of your personality you like, the parts of your physical appearance that you can appreciate, the reasons why you're a good person, your knowledge, your experiences, and the challenges you've overcome. This will feel difficult, but push through it. Ask someone you love to help if you get stuck.

Become the Loving Parent

It may surprise you (or cause you to roll your eyes) to read that almost all your anxious beliefs and feelings come back to childhood in some way. Even if you didn't notice anxiety in yourself until more recent times, and even if you consider yourself to have had a healthy, happy childhood, there's still a scared little child in you yearning for your attention.

For example, the anxiety you feel as an adult around your partner potentially leaving you might stem from the pain of being left by a father who wasn't very consistent in your early life. The pressure you feel to produce high-quality work all the time might come from having a parent who celebrated you based on your grades in school and always pushed you to be the best. Never being able to sit quietly and relax might come from having a mother who always told you to just keep yourself busy when you were upset or bored as a child. The experiences we have early in life can set us up for anxiety later on, even when our parents had the best intentions.

We all have a part of us, the inner child, hoping for that parent to give us their praise or approval. Our inner child still yearns to hear a parent say something like "I am proud of you. I'm so glad I'm your parent. You're a great kid. I love you. You're so important to me." This occurs even for those of us with parents who were attentive and loving, as well as for those whose parents did not meet their needs. Each of us has experienced a moment when our parent couldn't reassure us with exactly what we needed to hear. As small children with undeveloped emotional maturity, we couldn't communicate what we needed.

The good news is that it doesn't matter what kind of childhood experiences you had, or whether you had supportive, loving parents or unstable parents. Now that you are an adult, you have the ability to become the most healing, wonderful loving parent to yourself. Only you know exactly what you need to hear to feel loved and safe. Only you know what you require moment to moment.

Start to see yourself as having two parts: your loving parent and your inner child. Your loving parent is your true, loving self and your inner child is your fear-based anxious mind. Whenever you're afraid, worried, or upset, you also have a part of you that sees the scared little child and can bring it love and support.

Becoming the loving parent might look like taking some time to listen to yourself, the way you always wanted to be heard, and speaking out loud or writing down your worries and concerns. It could be holding space for yourself to break down and cry. It might look like physically wrapping your arms around yourself. You might place a hand on your breastbone for a feeling of support. It could be speaking words of kindness, love, and praise to yourself, saying to yourself those words you've always wished someone else would tell you. You could say, "I'm here for you now. I'm with you. You don't have to do this alone. I love you as you are. I love you unconditionally and you never have to earn that. You matter to me, and I'll always be here."

You could spend your whole life waiting to hear your mother or father say these words to you. In many cases, they never will. And even when they do, can they ever say it enough? Will they say it every time you need it? It's time to see you don't need to wait around for the perfect parents to move on with your life and help that little child within you feel safe and loved. You can give the praise you always wanted to hear to yourself right now. You can give yourself everything you always needed. This isn't about being hyper-independent and never needing another human being. If there's anything you feel you can't give to yourself on your own, understand that you have the means to go and get that support. You have a voice to ask for help, you can learn new skills, you can gain knowledge, and, in this way, you have the ability to acquire all the resources you'll ever need. That is a very empowering mindset indeed.

Mental Notes

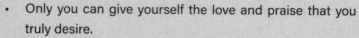

- Only you can give yourself the love and praise that you truly desire.
- At some point you just have to decide to start backing yourself and giving yourself everything you always needed by becoming your own loving parent.

Practice

What words have you always wanted to hear from your parents? Can you give them to yourself today? Practice bringing in the loving-parent part of you next time you're feeling anxious, stressed, or upset. Use your words and hug yourself or place your hand on your heart.

My clients often tell me this practice is really difficult. If you feel the same, I urge you to question that. It's hard to learn another language. It's hard to climb Mount Everest. Is it really hard to sit where you are right now in your comfortable home and just give yourself a hug? Is it really hard to speak some words out loud? Question your resistance to this and keep going, because the resistance you feel is actually a clear indication that this is the healing you most need to move forward.

Stimulants and Depressants

You may be aware that consuming certain substances such as coffee and alcohol can have an impact on the level of anxiety you experience. Or perhaps you don't believe there are any anxiety-inducing consequences for you. You may well be surprised at what I have to share. Here, we explore how and why sipping some of your favorite beverages may be drilling a hole in your Resilience Shield.

Caffeine Is Anxiety Fuel

I have never been much of a coffee drinker. A few years ago, I said yes to the offer of a free soy latte at a conference, to keep my mind stimulated so I could absorb all the rich, valuable information the speakers were sharing. I was feeling a little sleepy after sitting still and without any natural light for so long. Within minutes of ingesting the delicious coffee, my heart was beating uncomfortably fast and my hands were shaking to the point of turning my previously neat notes into scribble, as though I'd written them drunk. I did feel the kickstart in my brain and the edge to my focus, so the other side effects were manageable. It felt somewhat worth it, until that night as I lay awake, exhausted yet unable to sleep until 2 a.m. That's what coffee and other high doses of caffeine do to my body, without fail, every time.

While not everyone's body responds with the same intensity, I know many of you reading this will be nodding your head at my story here. Even if you think your body handles caffeine pretty well and you don't get the jitters, there is no doubt it is still affecting your sleep quality, which in turn affects your anxiety. Sometimes we just aren't aware enough to notice what a coffee or more a day is doing to our anxiety.

Caffeine is anxiety fuel. Coffee is the most popular beverage in the world, and it contains around 95 milligrams per cup—though coffee is not the only source of caffeine we consume. There's caffeine in black tea (47 milligrams); green tea (30 milligrams); chai tea lattes (40 milligrams); and dark chocolate, cocoa, cola beverages, and pre-workout supplements (ranging from 150 to 400 milligrams per serving). Even decaf coffee isn't totally decaffeinated; you will still consume up to 20 milligrams of caffeine per cup.

Excessive caffeine consumption typically leads to heart palpitations, a fast heartbeat, tremors, shaking, agitation, and restlessness. (Sounds a lot like anxiety.) Just take a moment to consider what that caffeine intake might be doing to your body in terms of overloading your already frazzled nerves.

Now, just so you know I'm not just pulling facts out of thin air, there is evidence that caffeine consumption increases stress hormone levels—namely cortisol.[2] This happens for any human being drinking coffee, no matter your tolerance level or genetics. Caffeine is spiking cortisol levels and stressing out our bodies more than necessary.

What if we combine caffeine consumption with mental stress? The rise in stress hormones is amplified. Let's say, for example, Sally is at work and she's having a really busy day. She has a ton of emails to respond to. Then her boss walks in with another task saying, "Oh, and by the way, I need this done by the end of the day." Sally is already stressed out, and now she's feeling added pressure. Her stress hormones will naturally rise in such a situation, and because she had coffee that morning, the rise is even greater than it would have been without caffeine in her system. Considering that most of us live in high-pressure environments with great demands on us, and many of us drink coffee to help us keep up with these demands, this magnified rise in cortisol is happening all too commonly.

When we combine exercise with caffeine, such as taking a pre-workout supplement before a gym class, the rise in cortisol is also exaggerated. This is in contrast to exercise without caffeine in the system, which does not alter cortisol levels and can help us better cope with stress and anxiety.

Trust me: If you're reading this book, your body already has enough stress hormone triggers to deal with. It does not need the added kick caffeine provides.

I encourage you to reflect on this. Have you ever had a break from coffee or the other sources of caffeine mentioned here? Have you ever pushed past the first week or more, so that you can experience the improvement in your sleep quality and energy levels? Are you having trouble sleeping now? If so, it's a great idea to remove caffeine from your body for a period of time. I suggest starting with two weeks as your goal, and extending from there if you notice a difference.

Mental Notes

- Caffeine is fuel for anxiety, increasing levels of stress hormones in your body.
- Caffeine may be impacting your sleep quality, even if it doesn't directly make you feel more anxious.

Alcohol and Anxiety

Alcohol is a depressant, not a stimulant, but it has its own detrimental impacts on anxiety. Each of us has different levels of brain chemicals called neurotransmitters that impact how quickly our brain cells fire and the stability of our mood. Neurotransmitters such as GABA and serotonin are a key factor in regulating the physiological process that occurs in your brain as you experience anxiety.

Alcohol alters the levels of these calming neurotransmitters in the brain. While there appears to be a relaxing effect when you consume alcohol, it's lulling you into a false calm here. As soon as you sober up and the alcohol leaves your system, you're left with a kind of rebound effect of more anxiety. Anxiety is a very common symptom of a hangover. The alcohol essentially overstimulates the GABA receptors on cells in your brain as it behaves similarly to calming GABA. Yet overuse of alcohol can lead to ongoing desensitization of the GABA receptors on cells, meaning that it's harder for your brain to respond to the levels of GABA naturally present in your brain. Alcohol is literally making it more challenging for you to relax on your own.

Occasional use of alcohol is something most of us can bounce back from as long as we are prepared and learn to anticipate that the cost of drinking will include a day or two of anxiety afterward as we recover. It is not necessary to never drink alcohol again, but you must understand the cost. It's far preferable to maintain a healthy social life than stop drinking altogether and never socialize. Simply bring some awareness to your intake and how it is affecting your mental health. It's also a good idea to stop drinking for a period of time while you work deeply on your anxiety, as this will really help you to reset your physiology.

Regular, habitual drinking is another story and can further numb the brain to its own calming chemicals. The effect is more significant and long-lasting, though with support you can recover the functioning of your brain after alcohol abuse. Habitual drinking is akin to overloading the brain with a calming substance (the alcohol), and then your brain has trouble regulating itself on its own when the alcohol is no longer there.

Think of anyone you know in your life who is a heavy drinker. When they're not on the booze, they are probably anxious. If you've noticed your alcohol consumption is creeping up—if you're frequently using alcohol to unwind at the end of the day or to get to sleep—it's time to get really honest with yourself and confront this habit. It needs to change if you're going to get control of anxiety.

A Note on Pharmaceutical Drugs

It may surprise you to learn that many pharmaceutical drugs come with anxiety as a side effect. For example, a number of migraine medications contain caffeine. Corticosteroids—which are often used to treat rheumatoid arthritis, inflammatory bowel disease, asthma, allergies, and many other conditions—mimic cortisol in the body and may cause anxiety. Other examples include medications used for thyroid disease, attention-deficit hyperactivity disorder (ADHD), and epilepsy. Importantly, some of the most common side effects of selective serotonin reuptake inhibitor (SSRI) medications, which are often used to treat anxiety, include nervousness, restlessness, and agitation. Anxiety is very common upon withdrawal from these medications. Please note that this information is for educational purposes and not medical advice. You must check with your doctor if you suspect your medication may be contributing to your anxiety, as stopping a prescribed medication without the supervision of your doctor can be dangerous.

Your At-Home Experiment

If you've never completely removed caffeine from your body for a period of time, you can't know for sure the kind of impact it is having. The same is true for alcohol. You may also require deeper support if any of these substances have become your coping mechanism for anxiety.

There are alternatives that can help to ease the transition as you reduce your intake of caffeine and alcohol. You can consume sparkling water with lemon, experiment with mocktails, or try flavored kombucha drinks to still feel like you're a part of the drinking ritual with friends. When it comes to replacing the soothing, comforting cup of coffee, there are many options to consider. If you have a search in your local health food store or online, you'll find roasted dandelion root coffee alternatives and medicinal mushroom-based latte powders that taste delicious.

Practice

Do you notice that caffeine has an impact on your sleep or anxiety? If yes, it's time to start tapering off your caffeine intake and ideally remove it completely.

Have you ever had a complete break from caffeine? If no, it's time to take a break now.

Is your alcohol intake creeping up? Are you using it to manage your anxiety? If yes, it's time to address this issue in your life and reduce your consumption or take a break completely.

When did you last have a long-term break from alcohol? If you can't remember, now is the time to take a break.

Please note, you may reintroduce these substances later on, but note how you feel as you do so. You can then make an informed choice about what is best serving you from there.

Week Two Checklist

You have six practices to work with in your second week. Revisit the sections earlier in this chapter for the full details. You might find some of the practices challenging to work through. Embrace these challenges as exciting opportunities to grow!

☐ Make a guess about the messages your anxiety commonly tries to bring you.

☐ Take note of the coping mechanisms you use to numb or distract yourself from anxiety.

☐ Journal your responses to the questions for each basic mental health need.

☐ Write a two-page self-love letter.

☐ Practice being your own loving parent by speaking the words you need to hear when you feel anxious.

☐ Take a two-week break from caffeine and alcohol. Note and evaluate how this makes you feel.

Week Three: Believing It Can Change

Asking for More

If you take a moment and close your eyes, what would your dream life look like? How good could it get for you? So often the anxious mind fantasizes about the worst-case scenario and how bad it could get. Let's challenge that. What if you had all the resources you needed? What would you be doing with your life? What would your work life look like if you could choose? How would your relationships be different? What about having wealth and abundance beyond what you need? What would it feel like to have optimal health and energy? How would it feel to have a limitless mind? What would it take for you to call your life wonderful? What does your heart yearn for?

Take the vision you've just created, and double it. Why did you stop there? What if it could get even better than that? Even if it seems like a long shot, just allow yourself to enjoy the free feeling of dreaming and letting your imagination wander, like you did when you were a child.

Notice how just allowing yourself to ponder these questions creates a palpable change in your body? This is because it changes your state of mind into one that feels expansive. An expanded state of mind will always feel calm, exciting, free, and more loving, because this is much closer to the wavelength of your true self. It's taking you out of the limited-thinking, anxious mind. If you ranked yourself as low in your basic mental health need for more freedom in your life, this is one way you can work on it.

Now, I'd like you to ask yourself why you're not living your dream life now. What are the reasons? Be as honest as you can. As you come up with your list, you're hitting the gold. These are your limiting beliefs. They are thoughts about your circumstances and yourself that you've repeated so many times, you believe they are true.

Right now, you are likely telling yourself a story about you. It might go something like this: "I'm an anxious, high-strung person. I've always been this way and I always will, because everyone in my family is like this and it's all I've really known. I'm a sufferer of anxiety, a victim of mental illness. I think there's something wrong with me, because I'm so weak willed and I self-sabotage all the time. I never follow through on what I start."

You'll also have decided that you have particular defining roles that you must fulfill: "I'm a mother, a daughter. I have to be a good partner. I'm a good person and a good student. I set a good example. I am a caregiver, a boss, an employee."

You might have decided you have (or lack) certain talents and skills. You have quite likely set a limit on your earning potential. Perhaps you've decided that you don't really deserve love, or maybe it just can't happen for someone like you. You may well be telling yourself the story that *they* can have it, but you can't. That you were born into a disadvantaged family situation that limits you, or one so privileged that you dare not ask for more—you should be more grateful. You might believe that because you have kids, you can't do anything you want to do, or that you have to stick with your current job, and it's your only possible income stream.

Am I reading your mind? That's because I've believed all these things too, and so have my clients. This is the sound of your anxious mind-stream undercurrent, and it is keeping you stuck in a less-than-fulfilling life. It's not about having billions of dollars and living on a yacht. It's about feeling that such an impossible life might be possible for you if you truly wanted it, if your mind would allow it. The feeling of possibility, openness, and expansion is what I'd love you to experience.

I've had clients go from anxious and miserable, being bullied at work and feeling undervalued, to starting their own businesses, working for themselves on their terms, selling their art, and quitting their corporate jobs. I've watched women upturn the unfair power dynamic at home in which they come last to one in which Mom is taken care of as well as the kids and partner. I saw one woman go from having daily panic attacks and being unable to leave home without her essential oil roll-on and phone in hand, just in case, to empowered and turning over $1 million in her business within twelve months. I've helped people who were exhausted from bloating and horrible digestive pain, given no answers from the gastroenterologist, scared that they'll never get their life back, and feeling like a shell of who they once were. I've watched these people heal their gut and master their anxious mind, bouncing back with a whole new mission in life to help others do the same. I saw a woman stuck in a cycle of daily binge drinking quit alcohol completely and come back to being present, loving, and patient with her little girls. I've witnessed women in abusive relationships discover their power and courage to leave, and fall in love with new partners who worship them. I've seen people so burned out, anxious, and unwell that they couldn't even leave their bed or get food down become filled with energy and love for their lives.

It's time to start romanticizing your life—seeing it like a book or a movie, in which you are the hero of your own story. Is your present chapter where a story would naturally end? No, the main character is about to overcome those obstacles in front of them, learn new things about themselves, and find their happy ending. And I'm rooting for that person, cheering them on. I want to see them win. Don't you? Of course, life works as an ongoing process of falling down, rising back up, and feeling empowered in that happily-ever-after moment, then falling down again as the next challenge arises. But if, during the most difficult times, you can keep an awareness that the next happy-ending phase is on its way, the down moments won't feel so hard.

So where do you want your story to go from here? What if you're the one who breaks the pattern of stress and anxiety and reaches for a life you never dreamed possible?

Mental Notes

- Asking for more changes your state of mind into one that feels expansive and open.
- Questioning your limiting beliefs shifts you out of the fear-based mind and aligns you back with your loving true self.

Practice

Get your journal out and write down the thoughts this chapter has inspired:

- What would your dream life look like?
- What is the story you are telling yourself about who you are? Where are you limiting yourself? Where are you playing life small? Why is that?

Aligning with Your Values

Do you know what your values are in life? For a long time I had no idea, and I didn't really understand the point in defining them. It was just something people talked about a lot in the self-development world. I've since come to learn that knowing your values is incredibly useful and it's a tool I now use with every client.

A value is simply something that is important to you. As you can imagine, values are different for everyone. Anxiety often offers a warning sign that your life is moving further away from what you value. This is a common reason for waking up with a feeling of dread about the day, or a sense that life is lackluster and unful-filling. Getting clear on your values will help you make sound decisions about the way you are living your life, so you can stay in close alignment with what you value. Knowing your values also helps you transcend the belief systems you may have inherited from your parents or other authority figures in your life. For example, your parents might have valued hard work, but hard work isn't as important to you as making a difference in somebody's life. When your life is aligned with your values, you will feel more grounded and authentic, and much less anxious.

The culture we live in tells us every day that success and happiness are found in the way we look, the things we have, and the material, external world. But the more we focus on material values, the more anxious we feel. It's so easy to focus on the surface-level things such as the shoes you wear, the shape of your eyebrows, the old car you drive, the number on the scale, or the likes on your social media account. But no one thinks about the incredible sports car or amazing shoes they own on their deathbed. What's truly important isn't material or external. It's the people we love, the lives we touch, the moments we feel we are truly living, freedom, things that stir our hearts, and the deeper, more fulfilling aspects of life. You must remind yourself where true happiness and success lies, and what's actually important to you. When you examine your values, you have an opportunity to prioritize the things that lift you out of anxiety and fear, and into a meaningful life.

Mental Notes

- Your values are a compass that can help you orient closer to where you feel best in your life.
- Whenever you need to make an important decision, coming back to your values will help bring you clarity. Simply ask: Which choice brings me more into alignment with what matters most?

Practice

Take a moment to consider the people in your life that you know, and those you don't know but admire and respect. They might be authors, presenters, politicians, scientists, influencers, or actors. Who inspires you? Make a list.

Now consider the reasons why they invoke this feeling in you. What is it about them that grabs your attention and your heart? Is it the way they conduct themselves with self-love? Is it the freedom you see in their lifestyle? Is it their authenticity? Is it the way they treat others? You'll start to see some common themes. See if you can come up with a list of values for yourself, based on these things you admire in others.

Some examples of values include: kindness, freedom, authenticity, respect, love, connection, vulnerability, being of service, abundance, success, flow, spirituality, connection to nature, resilience, family, relationships, purpose, contribution, openness, growth, loyalty, honesty, courage, generosity, selflessness, empowerment, altruism, self-reliance, empathy, and determination.

Finally, consider your top values and ask yourself how closely you are living in alignment with these values.

The next step will be clear. What needs to change?

Finding Your Purpose

You've experienced the feeling of dreaming your heart's biggest desires. You've connected to your values. If you're feeling unclear about your purpose in life, it's now time to put these two together. What was it that you loved doing as a child? When were you happiest? Were there certain activities you engaged in or behaviors you exhibited that you just did because they felt good?

Charlie was burned out, lost, and unclear about his purpose. He was thinking of quitting his healthcare clinic business and starting all over again. It all seemed so pointless to him. I asked Charlie to relax with his eyes closed, and I guided him through a hypnotherapy process in which he went back to what he loved doing as a child. Closing our eyes allows us to better access our subconscious mind, so we can gain deeper insights. You can try this too. I asked him to connect to that feeling of childlike joy and describe the memories that came up. I learned that as a child, he was often in the garden. It was a pleasure to plant seeds and follow his curiosity about the different varieties of flowers and vegetables. He loved watching the seedlings grow under his watchful nurturing and guidance. It brought such delight and a feeling of connection to the wider environment around him. He felt valuable, like he was having an impact on the world.

Bogged down in the menial administrative tasks of running his clinic day to day and managing his own patients was a far cry from the guiding, connected, and impactful feeling his heart was longing for. After we explored his younger self's passions, we reframed Charlie's perspective on his business and highlighted some key changes that would help. He stepped back from the administrative tasks he found so draining, passing them on to a receptionist. He reduced his patient-facing days. He took on a more overseeing, guiding role. From this place, he had more time to learn and guide the business from a leadership position. He could see the wider impact his business was having on the community around him, tend to its growth, and appreciate the progress he was making. He learned to view his business like a garden he was taking care of. Suddenly work felt exciting and fulfilling again. He reconnected with a deep sense of purpose.

As you can see from Charlie's story, sometimes the connection between your childhood passions and your adult life is not literal; in fact, often it's not. It's about noticing the overarching themes in what you used to love—such as being connected to a community or creating things with your hands. If you loved playing with animals, you don't have to become a vet. You could become a breeder, adopt a pet, volunteer at an animal shelter, become a dog trainer, or work at the zoo. Or maybe it is as simple as working in a dog-friendly coworking space. If you enjoyed sports, ask yourself what elements of sports you loved. Was it moving your body and feeling free, or was it the feeling of being part of a team?

As a child I was always happiest exploring my imagination, drawing pictures, and playing in nature, so I integrate those things into my life now. It still blows my mind that I get to go out walking on clifftops overlooking the beach and take video footage to turn into inspiring social media content. As I walk, breathing in the ocean air, I drift off into my imagination, putting ideas together for new podcast episodes or book chapters. As a young person I also naturally enjoyed being of service: helping my brother find the pieces he needed as we built LEGO cities together, and never eating a freshly baked treat from my grandmother without splitting it with my siblings. I love sharing joy with others. When I go without these things in my life for too long, anxiety will soon remind me of their importance.

Practice

Let's clarify your purpose. What did you most love doing as a child? What were the elements of that activity that brought you joy? Was it the collaboration and connection with people? Was it being creative, drawing, painting, or dreaming up stories and ideas? Could it have been organizing information and coming up with plans? Was it using technology, or being out in nature? Was it helping people and sharing? What about using your hands or playing with numbers?

Write down any ideas you have about your purpose. If it isn't clear to you just yet, remain open to the idea that inspiration will find you. You might also ask: What inspires my curiosity? What people, places, and activities energize me? And how can I bring more of those things into my life?

Don't give up if the answers don't come to you immediately. Instead, encourage yourself by saying, "I'm on my way to figuring out my purpose and I'm open to new ideas and solutions."

Activating the Vagus Nerve

Did you know that you have a built-in anxiety off switch? This is a section of the book to return to whenever you'd like a selection of quick and easy tools to move you out of an anxious state and into a state of feeling grounded and calm. We have arrived at the first part of the optimal gut health component of the Resilience Shield. Allow me to introduce you to your vagus nerve.

First, you need to understand how the nervous system works. It's a complex collection of nerves and neurons. These act like electrical wires in your body and are responsible for the activated, anxious feeling you have when you're triggered by a stressful thought or scenario. Some of these wires have a voluntary, under-your-control response. They're part of the somatic nervous system and the reason you can move your limbs, dance, and talk. The rest of the wires are involuntary, and they respond automatically without your conscious input. They keep your breathing going, your blood flowing, and your digestive system moving without you thinking about it. This is the autonomic (think "automatic") nervous system. The autonomic nervous system operates in two modes: sympathetic and parasympathetic.

The sympathetic nervous system controls your fight-or-flight response. In this state, the blood flow in your body moves predominantly to your limbs, so that you are ready to run away from danger or fight if need be. Your breathing becomes faster and your digestive system shuts down. You don't need to be digesting food in an emergency. It's all about survival. In the past, fight or flight was incredibly useful for getting away from a predator once in a while or responding to a rare near-death moment. But nowadays, many of us are living in this survival state every day, for many hours of the day. Every anxious thought, every stressful work email, every confrontational conversation with a friend, every incoming message you need to respond to, every horrible news story, every glance at your unending to-do list, and every traffic jam or near-miss collision sends the sympathetic nervous system firing into action.

You can imagine how living in this chronic activated emergency mode leads to gut problems, because your digestive system either stops moving altogether or it moves your food through too quickly. (Hello constipation or diarrhea. Or both.) There's not enough blood flow to properly absorb your nutrients and the whole system is unable to break down your food optimally. When you're in an emergency, the last thing the brain cares about is making babies, so you'll often have hormone imbalances and reproductive health issues over time as well. Your sleep cycle, skin health, thyroid status, liver function, and immune system are all affected.[1]

You can't avoid stress and anxiety altogether. They're a part of life. However, there's no doubt that switching out of a sympathetic nervous system state more of the time is a huge win for your overall well-being, as well as your experience of anxiety.

The parasympathetic nervous system is where you're aiming to be. This system is commonly called rest-and-digest mode. This is where your body is relaxed, so blood flow moves to your abdomen. Your breathing slows down and your digestive system is active and working well to break down and digest your food. Your reproductive system also receives a lot more attention, with the hormones that control your menstrual cycle flowing in an orderly, balanced fashion that keeps period problems at bay and your fertility health optimal.

Now back to the vagus nerve. Think of your vagus nerve as the on switch for the parasympathetic nervous system and the off switch for the sympathetic nervous system. It runs all the way from your brain to your gut, connecting your mental state to your digestive system. If your mouth is producing saliva, you have activated your vagus nerve. If you're hungry and feel your stomach rumbling for food, you're in rest-and-digest mode. If you're feeling calm and relaxed, your parasympathetic nervous system is working. You can use the vagus nerve to deactivate the sensation of anxiety, like a light switch. You can also strengthen this process, so it happens more often and becomes your natural home state, by activating the vagus nerve regularly. This is called toning the vagus nerve, and it's much like toning muscle. An understanding of the processes that activate and tone the vagus nerve is a very useful tool to have up your sleeve. You can activate your vagus nerve anywhere, any time, whenever you need.

There are countless ways to activate your vagus nerve, but here you'll find my favorites that will weave seamlessly into your lifestyle.

Bitter Foods

Eating bitter foods makes your mouth tingle, stimulating your salivary glands and activating your digestive system. Salivation is one of the first steps of the digestive process, and if your digestion is activated, so is your parasympathetic nervous system. Examples of bitter foods include lemon juice, sauerkraut, endive, rocket leaves, kale, parsley, and apple cider vinegar.

Apple Cider Vinegar Shot

Taking a shot of apple cider vinegar about fifteen minutes before you eat breakfast is a great way to set yourself up for a calmer, more relaxed day. Always dilute your apple cider vinegar with water at a ratio of one part apple cider vinegar to two parts water. Imagine a standard shot glass. Fill one third with apple cider vinegar (approximately 5 milliliters) and two thirds with water (approximately 10 milliliters). That should give you an idea of a good amount to aim for.

The effect on your nervous system is not dose dependent, meaning you can achieve the same result with a tiny drop of vinegar on your tongue; more will not produce a stronger effect. If you're worried about your tooth enamel, throw the shot to the back of your mouth. You can also switch out apple cider vinegar for lemon juice if you prefer. It works much the same. The trick is to not drink an entire glass of water with your lemon juice or apple cider vinegar as this will dilute the bitter taste too much and will also dilute your stomach acid, leading to weaker digestion. (I always recommend avoiding drinking a lot of liquid with meals, waiting around twenty minutes either side for optimal digestion.)

Legs Up the Wall

You can activate your parasympathetic nervous system by lying down with your legs up the wall for fifteen to twenty minutes. You may have tried this posture in yoga. Your body will take on an L-shape, with your torso flat against the ground and your legs resting up as vertically as you can get them. This practice works well in the evenings, calming your nervous system and preparing you for sleep. The L-shaped position works by using gravity to send the blood flow from your legs to your abdomen, mimicking the rest-and-digest state of the body. It naturally increases the production of GABA, that key calming chemical in your brain, which we'll discuss in more detail later on in this book.

Deep Belly Breathing

Place one hand on your chest and one hand on your belly. Don't change your breathing yet; just take a few breaths and notice where your breath is naturally more dominant. When you're in fight-or-flight mode, the breath sits higher up in the chest. This type of breathing is also called prey breathing, because it is quiet and shallow—like that of a rabbit or deer hoping to remain undetected by a predator. It sends a message to your brain to remain on high alert. Taking deeper, longer, and louder breaths deep into the belly, and even sighing out on your exhale, will bring you into rest-and-digest mode, activating the parasympathetic nervous system.[2] You might like to incorporate deep belly breathing into your morning meditation, just before you go to sleep at night while your legs are up the wall, or whenever you are waiting at a traffic light. It can help to position little reminders throughout your day to breathe, so you can keep it up automatically and consistently. Taking five to ten deep breaths into your belly once or twice daily is a great practice. You'll start to notice when you are breathing up high in your chest, and with that awareness you can bring your breathing back down into your belly.

Chanting "Om"

Your vagus nerve responds to your vocal cords' vibrations. The traditional yoga chant of the word "om" activates the vagus nerve. Researchers studied the effect of "om" chanting in bus drivers, with bus driving known to be a particularly anxiety-inducing job. Chanting almost daily over four weeks reduced their anxiety symptom scores, with the vibration affecting the vagus nerve and triggering the parasympathetic nervous system.[3] You can try this by chanting the "o" sound for about five seconds, followed by the "m" for as long as your breath can produce the sound. You'll always hear me loudly and proudly chanting "om" before and after a yoga class, knowing it's an added bonus for my nervous system. You can of course do this in the privacy of your own home or in your car when you need to ground yourself. Repeat it three to five times.

Cold Water Therapy

A quick shock of cold water for thirty seconds at the end of your usual hot shower will stimulate the vagus nerve and produce a relaxing effect afterward. You can even get the desired effect by splashing your face with cold water at the bathroom sink. You don't have to enjoy the experience of cold to enjoy cold water therapy. It's all about your mindset: do the uncomfortable thing and sit in that difficult moment, knowing it will soon be over and you'll feel really good. You'll feel proud of yourself knowing you did it—you chose to be with a feeling that most people would shy away from.

If you don't feel the effect after thirty seconds, try a little longer. I really like this technique to break an anxious thought cycle when you feel like you can't get out of your own head. It brings you straight back into the present moment and into your body.

Laughter

Similar to chanting "om," laughing also activates the vagus nerve, with emerging research suggesting that using laughter as a therapy can help decrease anxiety.[4] What do you need to set yourself up for more laughter in your day? Is it time with particular friends who make you laugh? A TV show you love? Letting yourself laugh out loud at a funny video on social media? Or just choosing to look for more things to laugh about in your day? You might be surprised at how you can bring out your sense of humor just by setting the intention to do so.

Food

If you're eating a meal, your body will shift into rest-and-digest mode. This is actually one reason why comfort eating can make an effective temporary coping mechanism for anxiety. However, here we are referring to a mindful, balanced eating practice. When you eat in a calm environment, your brain registers the sight of incoming food, you salivate, you chew, and your digestive system is activated. Blood flow moves to the digestive system, which creates a state of relaxation. Of course, if you're always eating on the go while watching the news on TV, scrolling on social media, or walking between meetings, this won't work as well. Your body will be a little confused. Give your brain a chance to receive the message that you are eating a meal. Take a moment to engage with the ritual of eating. Look at your food, smell your food, notice the flavors and textures as you chew, and chew your food well before you swallow. This will allow the body to properly prepare for digestion and optimize the relaxing effect of eating.

Mental Notes

- The vagus nerve is your anxiety off switch, and it can be triggered using the methods starting on page 93.
- The parasympathetic nervous system is your rest-and-digest mode, where you want to live more of the time, instead of in the anxious fight-or-flight mode of the sympathetic nervous system.

Practice

Choose two of the vagus nerve activation practices to implement into your daily routine. You can of course incorporate more than two, but keeping it simple will mean you'll be able to stick with it rain, hail, or shine, and create a lifelong habit. In the Anxiety Reset Program, we begin with the apple cider vinegar shot each morning and legs up the wall each evening.

Week Three Checklist

I assigned you four practices to work with in Week Three. You may need to go back through the chapter to remind yourself of the steps involved.

☐ Describe your dream life in your journal, and note any stories you are telling yourself about who you are and why you need to play life small.

☐ Complete the exercise designed to help you uncover and define your values. Ask yourself how you might live in closer alignment with the values you listed.

☐ Clarify your purpose by writing in your journal, using the questions to guide you.

☐ Choose two of the vagus nerve activation practices to incorporate into your daily routine.

Week Four: Uncovering the Truth

The Four Pillars of the Anxious Mind

It's time to delve a bit deeper into the anxious mind to uncover its truth. There are four pillars of the anxious mind that, when understood, will help you create more awareness of thoughts for your Resilience Shield. Knowing these pillars will save you a lot of unnecessary anxiety as you will have the knowledge needed to outsmart your wily mind. When you understand how the mind works, it becomes easier to separate your true self from your fear-based thoughts that are so sneaky and easy to believe. You can find moments of peace in the relentless chaos of life.

Pillar One: The Mind Will Always Think

Your mind will always think, and trying to clear your mind to complete stillness is a waste of time and energy. A lot of people with high-functioning anxiety think they're not able to meditate properly. They believe there is something wrong with their mind because they can't shut it up. The truth is, no one can fully stop their mind from thinking. You can experience gaps between thoughts, but the next thought will always come. Instead, the goal is to observe the thinking mind and be indifferent to the stream of thoughts it creates. You can watch them pass by, without latching on to them or reacting too much to their content—no matter how scary, weird, or critical they might be. When you observe the mind, you have the ability to step away from those fearful, stressful thoughts and instead get curious about whether the thoughts are actually true. Most of the time, the fear is irrational and irrelevant to your current situation, adding no real value to your safety or love for yourself.

While you can't switch off your thinking, you can slow down your thinking. Your thinking will naturally slow down when you meditate and watch your thinking mind; when you activate your parasympathetic nervous system via the vagus nerve; and when you bring your awareness into your physical body.

Pillar Two: The Mind Will Always Find a Problem

The mind will always look for problems to solve and reasons to not feel peaceful in the moment. This is because the anxious mind is trying to help you survive, scanning the world around you for potential threats, problems, reasons to worry, and things that could go wrong. To the mind, there are never enough resources available to solve all the problems it can conceive. This is why it perpetually wants more: more money, more security, more love, and more experiences to quell its discontent. It is never satisfied, no matter what you do.

You have the ability to shift the focus of your awareness away from your thinking mind. You can recognize that finding problems and considering worst-case scenarios is just what the mind does. So when you next catch your mind doing this, you can notice what is happening and disengage. You can create space between you and the problem-finding mind and say, "Hey, mind! I'm on to you. I see what you're doing. You're just looking for problems right now and I don't have to follow along with you." In that moment you can awaken to the realization that you are, in fact, safe to focus on the task in front of you or the beauty of the world around you. This is available to you.

Pillar Three: The Mind Will Always Criticize

You will always have an inner critic. It's part of being human. There's nothing wrong with you if you notice your inner critic is back with a vengeance or it's speaking to you really loudly today, even after you've been working on using your loving-parent voice. You haven't gone backward. The goal of mastering your anxious mind is not to eradicate the inner critic. The goal is to let the inner critic operate as it will, and watch it with curiosity at a distance—not reacting to the irrelevant, boring content of its critical monologue. You're making progress if you notice that voice saying, "You idiot. How could you be so stupid?" and you let the statement be there, without taking it in. You watch the words go by, and you say, "That's my inner critic talking. I don't trust my inner critic. It never tells the truth. I'm not going to believe that."

Cultivate an awareness that the inner critic is an unreliable source of information. If the critical mind is spewing out judgmental, self-harming thoughts about you, chances are what it's saying isn't true. The inner critic is a misguided self-protection mechanism that is doing more harm than good. All through your life, your inner critic will extend a hand out toward you, inviting you to be unkind to yourself. Your job is to refuse the invitation as often as you can remember to. In doing so, you can turn down the inner critic's volume.

Pillar Four: The Mind Wants Control

Your mind is reacting normally to a big, chaotic, complicated life. It seeks control, and yet the external world is inherently out of control, unpredictable, and ever-changing. The mind wants the world to remain fixed, for everything to stay the same and be predictable. It wants the world to be unnaturally stable. This is what the mind does, because it is seeking safety in that control. You can become aware of this with compassion for yourself and what the anxious mind in you is trying to achieve, without blindly following it. Real control is always found in seeing through the predictable nature of the mind and choosing not to follow it.

It's time to stop complaining about the way the mind operates. It's time to stop rejecting and fighting against this uncomfortable part of yourself, finding more and more reasons to believe you are wrong and broken because you have a mind. It's time to realize that the anxious mind is only uncomfortable for you when you are totally unaware of how it works. The moment you become conscious and bring awareness to the mind's rules you begin to find a state of peace within. You don't have to buy into what your mind is doing or saying. You don't have to believe it or go along with it. You can step back and observe your thoughts.

True peace comes in the brief moments in which you realize you are so much more than your anxious mind. Perhaps you can feel that you are in one of those moments right now as you read these words.

Examining Your Thoughts

One of the most important skills you can develop in your life is the ability to examine your thoughts. When you question the way you think, you can honestly achieve whatever it is you want in your life. You can be whoever you want to be. If you leave your thoughts unexamined, though, you will automatically believe that whatever your mind produces is the truth. If the mind tells you that you are not the kind of person who finishes what they start, or that you are a quiet, shy person, you will take that as a true fact about you. But the real truth lies in understanding that you can decide what you want to tell yourself and believe as fact. Your mind is your loyal servant, and it will respond to what you tell it to think. When it comes to those seemingly impossible dreams you might have, if you think you can achieve them, you most likely can. If you think you can't, you can't. And you won't try. You get to decide which thoughts you want to keep thinking, and which you're going to start dismissing as irrelevant mind junk that you do not need to believe.

If you repeatedly think of yourself as a person who is unworthy of healthy relationships and exciting opportunities in life, what kind of emotions might come up for you? You'll likely feel less energized, deflated, and unmotivated. The actions you then take will be fueled by that emotion. When you feel apathetic and tired, you don't tend to take much action at all toward the results you want. You might not even have the energy to ask yourself what you really want. And so the results you get tend to prove that original thought true. You don't put the work in to attract and build fulfilling relationships, or even believe they're possible for you. You don't look out for those exciting opportunities, or put yourself in the situations that will bring them to you more easily, because why bother?

If you think that you're a wonderful human being, deserving of a life full of joy, love, and abundance, what do you think you are more likely to experience? Your eyes will be open, looking for these experiences, taking them in, and receiving them.

In my midtwenties I went through a phase in which I'd repeatedly come up with an exciting business idea, and spend weeks enthusiastically making plans and putting the concept together. I'd tell my friends and family (and anyone else who would listen) about my idea. Then my excitement would wane. I'd start to doubt the whole thing.

My mind created thoughts like "This is stupid. You don't know what you're doing. How is this even going to work? No one would want this." I would stop taking action on it and give up. I went through this pattern a number of times, feeling more and more disheartened.

One day, as I was journaling my thoughts, I became aware that I'd developed a belief around this. "I don't finish what I start" was the thought turning over and over in my mind. I believed that I would never be able to birth an idea fully into reality. As soon as I saw it for what it was—a story made up in my mind about who I am and what I'm capable of—I decided to change it. I started actively, repeatedly reminding myself of a new thought: "I'm the girl who gets it done. I make my dreams my reality." This thought felt empowering and exciting. It got me enthused to take action. I felt unstoppable.

Within a month I had come up with a new business idea. It was to create and sell a unique paste made out of fresh whole turmeric, honey, ginger, and spices that could be stirred into a hot cup of milk to instantly brew a delicious anti-inflammatory golden turmeric latte. I'd created a business plan, put the product together, taste-tested it with groups of people, hired a designer for the labels, applied for the necessary permits, found a commercial kitchen where I could make my paste, and started selling it in cafés around Melbourne. I got it done. I made it happen. This idea became a real product I could hold in my hands, a product that other people loved. And it all started with the way I influenced my mind.

Your mind responds to whatever you tell it. It is a tool that you can influence and steer in the direction that serves you best. It's time to challenge your thinking.

Mental Notes

- When you make it a priority to examine your thoughts, you unlock unlimited potential in your life to create your dreams.
- Your thoughts influence the way you feel, which dictates the actions you take. Your actions are what produce the results you have in your life.
- You get to choose which thoughts to allow in and accept as truth, and which thoughts to dismiss as useless, negative mind junk.

Practice

You've been working on becoming more aware of your thoughts; now let's start to question them. Write down your anxious, worrisome, fear-based thoughts for a few minutes. Start by writing, "What worries/scares me is..." and finish the sentence. Then, challenge each of the thoughts with the following questions:

- Is this really true?
- What if it isn't true?
- How does it make you feel to think this way?
- How could you think about it in a different way that makes you feel better?

Caring About What People Think

By default, your mind cares about what other people think of you—and you should be thankful it does. This is a very clever, built-in survival mechanism to ensure that when you're a vulnerable little child, you will remain a cohesive part of the family group you're born into. There will be other people there to help you acquire food, live safely under shelter, and find fresh drinking water, particularly at a time of life when you are unable to meet these needs on your own.

There is no need to pressure yourself to eradicate this element of your anxious mind completely. It's part of being human, after all. You simply need to understand why you care about what others think, bring awareness to it, and question the beliefs behind it. You can certainly learn to care a whole lot less about what other people think of you, but a part of you will always naturally sense for the feel of the group around you—what their needs are and how you can better get along with them. This is a good thing, because it means you can read people's emotions, understand them, and connect more deeply. Remember that connection and belonging is one of your basic mental health needs.

Of course, this mechanism can go too far. Caring too much about what other people think might manifest as social anxiety when you go to an event. Your mind might come up with all kinds of imaginary stories about how the other people there are judging you and the reasons why you don't fit in with them. You might feel an excessive need to edit your appearance, whether with makeup or social media filters, just so that others will like and accept you. You might choose a career path based on what would make your parents happy, or say yes to hosting the family at your house for the holidays when you'd rather not. You might think you have to say yes because everyone expects you to, and they'll be upset if you don't. You might frequently experience swirling doubt, worrying that you have overshared with a friend or offended someone because they haven't immediately replied to your text message.

To reduce the level of care you have for what others think of you, there are three key elements to consider: letting their stuff in, being vulnerable, and seeking others' approval.

Stop Letting Their Stuff In

Imagine you're driving your car home at night and, in the evening fog, you can't see clearly. Next thing, you've accidentally cut someone off. You've made a mistake, but no one has been hurt and no car has been damaged. Imagine that the person you've cut off is now having a road-rage moment, shaking their fist out the window and yelling at you aggressively. You can choose to perceive this scenario in two ways. You can believe this driver is attacking you because you are a bad person for not seeing their car and you deserve this punishment. You can beat yourself up, feel ashamed for messing up like you always do, and let those mean words in. Or you can choose to think a little more about it. You can put yourself in the other person's shoes and wonder with curiosity what would cause them to overreact. You can choose to see that this isn't really about you—that this person was somehow primed and ready to express anger today and it would have happened to anyone who crossed paths with them. You just happened to be in the firing line. Perhaps this person comes from a family in which anger is unhealthily demonstrated as a way to feel heard and respected. There are a million different reasons why a person might react to you with judgment, but it's never really about you.

This concept applies to your friends, family members, and people you work with. For example, if your boss is disappointed in you for needing an extension on a deadline because your workload is so heavy and the team is understaffed, that says a lot more about the pressure your boss might be feeling (and projecting onto you) than your value as a team member. We often experience these moments in our personal relationships, when a loved one criticizes us unfairly or lashes out when we've done little to provoke such an emotionally charged response.

Keep reminding yourself that people can't react in aggression or judgment toward you without feeling a state of unease within themselves. Happy, content people do not judge or find fault in others. They let them be as they are. People who feel insecure and unhappy in themselves will seek a sense of significance in judging another person. Take back your power by putting up an imaginary protective wall. Say to yourself, "I don't need to let that in. No, thank you. You can keep that." Take control by choosing to give others the benefit of the doubt. Assume it is not really about you and that the other person is having a bad day, because life is challenging and you never know what someone is going through. Perhaps the other person also has an anxious mind, and it could be spilling out all kinds of harmful untruths at any moment, just like yours can. It can even become a game to imagine what might be causing the other person to respond as they are, instead of automatically blaming yourself and searching for what you did wrong. Other people are always reacting from what they think is right from their perspective, life experiences, and unique set of values and beliefs. The critical thoughts they think are just as meaningless and irrelevant as your own.

When a situation inevitably arises in which you find yourself caring about what someone else thinks, make the decision right now to be resolute in your worthiness, knowing that this potential negative opinion can't have anything to do with you. That rude behavior, those excluding comments, that judgmental or negative energy is no longer something you'll accept in your life as deserved by you in any way. Trust that you are a good person—a flawed, beautiful human who is trying their best. Trust that you can live safely in a world where people judge others sometimes, because your own words to yourself have the most impact on you—and you have full control of them.

Take it one step further and consider what's going on for you the next time you find yourself judging someone. Why are you unable to see this person with compassion in this moment? Is it because they don't deserve compassion, or is it because you gain something from judging them? Maybe you feel important, or righteous, or you're playing out a familiar pattern that was demonstrated to you in childhood and that gives you a sense of belonging to your family group. This practice gives you an insight into the place anyone who judges you might be coming from. It may even allow you to feel compassion for the next person who judges you, knowing that they can't find acceptance or peace in this crazy life.

Your job is to live your life as close to who you truly are as often as you can, letting others judge you along the way, knowing their judgment is not your problem. The most important opinion of you will always be the opinion you have of yourself. That's where your true power lies.

Practice

Consider someone you have recently felt judgment toward. Why were you unable to see this person with compassion? What did you gain from judging them?

What kinds of stories are you telling yourself about what other people think of you? Consider your friends, close family members, acquaintances, and work colleagues.

Be Vulnerable

It's natural to feel uncomfortable being vulnerable with others, especially if it wasn't consistently safe to share your deepest emotions with your caregivers growing up. However, this is yet another protective mechanism of the mind: It's trying to stop you from being excluded from the tribe. Once you realize this, you can see it for what it is and rise above it. It often comes hand in hand with the belief that you are too much to handle, that no one can relate to you or understand the painful feelings you have. Interestingly, the more you refuse to be vulnerable with others, the more you prove the idea that you are alone in your experience to be true. You don't allow anyone to get close enough to test whether it might be a false belief.

To be truly vulnerable, you have to expose yourself in a way that makes you feel naked onstage. It never feels easy. It is the ultimate test of your fear of rejection. Your mind will always pop in to question you and try to get you to stop, or at least tone it down. To be vulnerable you have to say, "This is something I feel really ashamed about." You have to hold up a fragile piece of yourself that someone could theoretically reject or judge you for, and point at it directly, saying, "Look at this. I'm not hiding it anymore. Here it is. This is the real me." To show another person your shame can feel excruciating, and it will no doubt bring on anxiety.

However, if you move into the discomfort of this experience, something magic will happen. You'll create connection: deep connection—the kind you've been longing for your entire life. You'll find that people might like you even more because they can relate to you. They can see you, all of you, and it's a truly beautiful sight to behold. If you've ever seen another person in their vulnerability you will understand the beauty I'm talking about. When you take off your intimidating, protective mask of perfection and show your weak parts to another person, you exude a wholesome confidence that says you accept yourself. That you are not afraid to share these parts of your-self, despite it being difficult to do so.

Everyone has things that they are terrified to share with others—stories laden with shame and self-judgment. When you show someone else that this is okay—by shining a light on your own shame—you offer the most incredible gift to them. You open a door. You give them permission to be vulnerable too. You say, "It's okay, I've got stuff too. I don't like the stuff, but it's a part of my experience. Here's a bit of it. What about you?" The other person can accept the gift or decline it—that's up to them and a reflection of where they're at in their own journey of accepting themselves. The only people who won't be able to bear seeing your vulnerability or who choose to judge you for it are those who judge themselves most harshly. This is a big sign, saying, "I am way too insecure to show the shame that I have within me to anyone." Everyone has shame. Some people are ready to expose it, and others are not. Regardless, you should be proud of yourself for leaning into the discomfort of being vulnerable.

This doesn't mean you must be vulnerable with everyone you meet, within five seconds of meeting them. Be kind to yourself and go slowly. Start by choosing to share with those who have earned your trust, before moving on to audiences of strangers.

The most fascinating part of this is that while you might expect to be judged for being vulnerable, more often the opposite happens. Those who witness another person being vulnerable actually receive the act with awe. They think, "Wow, look at her. She's so brave to tell us that." Haven't you thought the same thing, seeing someone tell an emotional, heart-wrenching story about their life? Maybe you've felt that after reading some of my story—a story I've willingly chosen to share with all the strangers who come across this book. I can do this, because I know how powerful vulnerability can be. I know the treasure on the other side of the icky discomfort, the way it can impact people, help them feel seen and connected. Should you choose to accept this most incredible, thrilling assignment of exposing more of your shame to those who you feel have earned enough trust to receive the gift of your vulnerability, you will reap the rewards. You will experience a deeper sense of connection and belonging than you ever thought was possible. You will create family out of friends, and friends out of family. Vulnerability is the secret to building beautiful relationships in your life, and lovingly accepting yourself more and more as you go.

Mental Notes

- Being vulnerable will always feel uncomfortable, but it is worth it for the deeper connections you'll create.
- Other people will perceive your vulnerability as bravery and naturally feel closer to you.

Stop Seeking Others' Approval

Feeling liked and having others' approval sends a signal to your brain to say that you're accepted. You're safe here. But while it would be great to live in a world where everyone likes you, not everyone will. Many people will like you, but some will not. And it has nothing to do with you. Some people just don't feel like liking stuff in general, and they readily project that dislike onto anything they see.

It is not fun to be caught in the perspective of disapproval, looking for things to judge. It is much more fun to live your life actively seeking what you do approve of: things that bring you delight and pleasure and make you feel grateful. So let's take a moment to switch up the power imbalance here and realize that anyone who does not approve of you is not having a fun time in their life. That's a shame for them, but you can't do anything about what they do. Those people get to go on disliking things, finding less and less joy in the process. You can only control what you tell yourself and where you choose to place your focus. Your challenge is to let them do what they want to do, and remember where the dislike is really coming from and what that means for their life experience. How great is it to see this now? You get to be aware of this and keep on finding things that you like about life and the people around you—and, of course, yourself.

The most important praise you will ever receive in your life is the praise that you give yourself. Use your loving-parent voice and imagine protective arms wrapping around you when you feel hurt that someone doesn't like you. Use it when you anticipate that others don't approve of you. Tell yourself the words you need to hear: that you're a worthy friend and a great person to be around; that you're lovable, kind, and caring; and that you have a lot to offer to the relationships in your life. Do this and you will care much less about what someone else thinks of you. In doing so, you will build more resilience to the anxiety provoked in social situations, and with family members, friends, partners, and so on. If you can approve of yourself, you won't spend your whole life waiting for someone else to do it for you. That's a very powerful place to be.

Mental Notes

- Some people just won't like you, and that's okay. Let them be in their unhappy, judgmental state.
- You don't have to wait around for someone to approve of you. You can give yourself all the praise and reassurance you've ever needed by practicing engaging with the loving-parent part of you.

The Gut and Anxiety

When Tess first reached out to me late one night with a message asking for help, she was feeling like a completely different person than who she had been two years before. The anxiety she'd developed was only getting worse. She was exhausted, with her sleep interrupted every night by fiery acid reflux and painful, bubbling bloating. She'd wake to the feeling of burning in her throat and was experiencing a constant, low-level panic. The doctor had referred her to a gastroenterologist who, after a series of invasive tests, couldn't give her any conclusive answers about what was going on. Instead, she'd been prescribed a cocktail of medications, none of which were providing relief. Tess was at a loss. She couldn't socialize with friends for fear of upsetting her stomach. She had to pull back to part-time hours at work and not even her beautiful new relationship could bring her joy. She was struggling to cope—frustrated and confused as to what step to take next.

After some further discussion, I learned that Tess was reacting with bloating and nausea to almost every food she ate, and she had completed several rounds of antibiotics over the previous two years due to recurring bladder infections. She was desperate to know what foods to eliminate next, but I knew the problem was not the food. It was the inflamed, raw state of her gut lining, sensitive like an open wound to almost any food she consumed. The gut–brain connection was a key root cause of her anxiety, and I was determined to embark on this journey with her to show her how powerful healing the gut could be in solving the distressing symptoms that had zapped her spark.

After three months of working together with a focus on gut healing, Tess did not return to being her old self, like she had first hoped when we began. She had instead grown into a completely new person, with renewed self-worth and a deep connection to her intuition. Her digestive symptoms had become entirely manageable and Tess now knew exactly how to listen to her body. Her sleep was consistent; her anxiety had been silenced. She was so inspired from her experience that she went on to start her own career helping other women empower themselves.

Let's start looking at how to optimize your gut health to create stronger resilience to the stresses of life and help your body relax. You don't have to have the same obvious and intense symptoms like Tess to experience the benefits of optimizing your gut health. Most of us have some degree of "leaky gut." Everyone can benefit from gut healing.

What Is the Gut?

Your gut is the entire tube running from your mouth to your stomach and right through to your anus, but usually this word is used to refer to the small and large intestines. We often forget that the gut is directly exposed to the outer world, just like your skin. It is the barrier between all factors external to your body and your internal organs, protecting them from invading pathogens, viruses, and bacteria, as well as wastes and toxins that should not be absorbed into your bloodstream.

The gut lining is the inner part of the tube that makes contact with the food you ingest. It acts as a wall of defense—a gateway to the bloodstream that determines what enters the body and what stays out. The gut lining is also home to the beautiful microbiome (more on that later). Every mouthful of food you eat has to be broken down and absorbed across the wall of the gut for those nutrients to flow into the rest of your body. As your gut contacts every system in the body, it plays an important role in regulating your immune system and maintaining healthy skin, energy levels, hormone balance, and levels of inflammation.

The Gut–Brain Connection

Your gut health has a key role to play in anxiety and your mood in general. This is mostly due to the gut microbiome, the vagus nerve, nutrient absorption, and its capacity to assist in regulating inflammation throughout the entire body. Beneficial bacteria from the gut microbiome can make chemical messages that are sent to the brain to balance out the brain chemicals that keep us feeling good, such as GABA, dopamine, and serotonin. While exact figures vary depending on the publication you're reading, it's said that around 95 percent of serotonin in the body is manufactured inside the gut.[1] However, the microbiome can easily fall out of balance, with invasions from pathogenic bacteria, overgrowths of healthy bacteria, or not enough beneficial species, making this process inefficient.

The brain has a profound impact on our digestive processes via the vagus nerve, as you've already learned. It disrupts digestive movement and cuts off blood flow to the digestive system if you are under stress. Many people experience loose bowel movements or constipation, or both, as a result of anxiety. Over time, this can develop into other digestion symptoms too, such as chronic bloating. Triggering the vagus nerve to activate the calming parasympathetic nervous system can turn this around.

An activated sympathetic nervous system can mean that nutrients are not effectively broken down and absorbed, as the bowels may be emptying too quickly for effective nutrient absorption to take place. This can create a deficiency in the nutrient building blocks required to make the calming brain chemicals in the first place, and the cycle goes on. You can eat the healthiest, most nutritious diet ever, and take all the supplements under the sun, but if your gut wall isn't in a state to absorb these nutrients, you won't experience much of an impact.

Lastly, inflammation in the brain at the microscopic cellular level leads to a number of problems with regulating feel-good brain chemicals. If there is inflammation in the gut there is inflammation in the brain.[2] By supporting and managing the leaky gut responsible for inflammation, the impact can be reversed. Knowing this information, you can use it to your advantage and build your mental health resilience from the gut.

What Is a Damaged "Leaky Gut"?

When working well, the cells of the gut lining sit neatly together and form a tight barrier that controls what gets absorbed into the bloodstream. A damaged, inflamed gut lining may contain cracks or holes between these cells, allowing partially digested food, wastes, toxins, and bacteria to penetrate the tissues beneath it without regulation. It's like gate-crashers sneaking past the bouncer at the party. This triggers an inflammatory response from the immune system, of which the gut wall houses an estimated 80 percent. The immune system is the next layer of defense, responding to the invading particles with an attack.[3] Every human has some degree of leaky gut. It isn't so much a diagnosable condition as a transient state that worsens with the typical stresses of modern life and improves with rest and a healthy lifestyle. The standard Western diet, which is low in fruits and vegetables and high in sugar, is a key contributor to leaky gut. Excessive (but socially accepted) levels of alcohol consumption, long stressful working hours, various medications and surgical procedures, and poor sleep habits—those things that define modern life—are the main drivers of gut inflammation.

How to Repair Your Gut Lining

There are two important steps to healing your gut lining, reducing inflammation, and managing leaky gut.

Step One: Remove Damaging Factors

Your gut has a natural ability to heal all on its own if you can remove as many damaging factors as possible from your diet and lifestyle. You can:

- limit alcohol and avoid recreational drugs
- limit processed foods high in sugar and other chemicals
- limit use of medications known to impact your gut health, such as the oral contraceptive pill, antibiotics, antifungals, and pain medications including nonsteroidal anti-inflammatories
- manage anxiety and stress by using the practices in this book
- prioritize adequate sleep, which is a key process for gut repair

Step Two: Repair

Next, you can provide the nutrient building blocks to repair tight junctions between the cells of your gut lining and reduce inflammation so repair can take place. I recommend these gut-healing foods:

- one cup of bone broth daily (contains both collagen and gelatine)
- one heaped tablespoon of collagen or gelatine powder daily
- turmeric, either added to your cooking or taken as a daily curcumin supplement

Collagen is an important protein that is found in almost every tissue in the body, including your gut lining. By increasing collagen intake from bone broth or collagen peptides, you can help support the lining of the digestive tract.[4] The most popular food to increase collagen intake is collagen peptides, a form of collagen that has been broken down so the amino acids can be more easily digested and absorbed. It can be added to hot drinks, tea, smoothies, and even cooked into soups, stews, and baked goods.

Bone broth is an ancient food that your great-grandparents likely consumed regularly. It is made by simmering bones, usually beef or chicken, for at least twenty-four hours to extract the nutrients and gelatine. These nutrients can facilitate the gut lining's healing process.[5] Bone broth can be used like stock as the base of many recipes, or consumed like miso soup as an afternoon snack.

Powdered gelatine is another option to increase collagen intake. It can be used to make jellies and gummies and to thicken sauces.

Turmeric, with its active components like curcumin, calms inflammation and actually switches on the genes that make your leaky gut sew itself back together.[6] These genes make more of the proteins that keep the cells close in a strong barrier, so that only the good things are absorbed and toxins, wastes, and pathogens remain out of your bloodstream.

Other important gut-healing nutrients include glutamine, zinc, and vitamin A. Work with a healthcare practitioner to ensure these are right for you before beginning a supplement regime. Medications, health conditions, pregnancy, and lactation are important to take into consideration. If you require a vegan or vegetarian option, my best advice is again to work with a healthcare practitioner to find a gut-healing supplement that suits your needs.

Practice

Begin by assessing your own gut health by answering the following questions:

- Is it usual for you to pass a bowel movement less than once per day?
- Is it usual for you to pass more than three bowel movements per day?
- Is your stool regularly loose, watery, or unformed?
- Do you experience digestive pain, unpleasant gas, or bloating more than once per month?

If you said yes to one or more of the aforementioned questions, you really could benefit from gut healing.

Next, start implementing the three gut-healing foods—bone broth, collagen/gelatine, and turmeric—or alternatives that suit you in your everyday routine.

Creating Certainty

Your brain thrives on predictability. Knowing your routine for the week means it can slip into autopilot and use up less energy to keep you safe. This is one reason so many people struggled during the pandemic: Suddenly their weekly routine was turned on its head. Every element of daily life changed in some way. Instead of leaving the house thinking, "Wallet, phone, keys," our brains had to learn the new routine: "Wallet, phone, keys, *face mask*." The routine of commuting to work became the unfamiliar experience of working from home, and many other life adjustments had to be made.

In recent times the uncertainty of life has never felt more apparent, and yet certainty is required for resilient, optimal mental health. Clients tell me, "I just want to know everything will be okay." How can you find a sense of safety, certainty, and stability despite the ever-changing, unpredictable world outside you? Don't despair. There is a way to create a sense of certainty, no matter what life throws your way.

First, you must ask yourself if you can see a clear vision of where you will be five years from now. Take a moment to pause and reflect before you read on. Do you know what your life will be like? Can you picture a scene of yourself going about your day?

It's completely fine if you can't see a clear vision. In fact, it's expected. You might be telling yourself that it depends on many factors. It depends on where you're living—if you end up in a different house, or a different city. It depends on whether you're still with your current partner, or single, or with a new partner. It depends on what role you're in at work, or whether your side business takes off. It depends on how much money you make. It depends on the state of your health. It depends on who is there, where you are, and what is happening around you. In other words, it all depends on your external environment.

If this is the case, you are living your life from a very conditional place. You're waiting for the external conditions to determine who you are and what your life looks like. It's here that you'll run into trouble, because there's no certainty in your career, your living situation, your finances, your marital status, or your love life. You can't rely on any of those circumstances to give you true stability. You will create so much stress if you need those circumstances to be fixed and certain. That's anxiety-inducing. You can drive yourself crazy waiting for everything to fall into perfect alignment in your life before you can feel safe. This is a rabbit hole down which you'll never find a satisfying, lasting sense of security. If you want to feel okay about your safety no matter what, you have to change your tactics.

The key is to take a look inside yourself to find certainty. What is it about *you* that is certain? What can you rely on in yourself? What can you be sure about in yourself regarding how you show up in the world, how you respond to challenges, and how you manage other people?

I'll give you an example. I know that no matter what happens, I have the ability within myself to create the meaning of my life. Even if my worst fears came true, I'd still find a way to make that circumstance serve me, somehow. It might take some time—maybe a year or two of processing the grief of the loss or change—but I know eventually I'll find a meaning that serves me. The hope and light in me cannot be broken. Some days it might feel more challenging; some days I may feel sad and need to cry. Ultimately, though, my true nature is being in a hopeful, loving, open state. I made that true for myself. I chose that identity and I repeated it over and over in my mind. I created certainty within me.

You can do the same. Let's practice creating true, lasting certainty within you.

Practice

Write down a list of five to ten personal qualities that you know to be true and certain about you—things that will be true even five or ten years from now. The aim is to develop a sense of knowing yourself deeply, so you can rely on aspects of yourself in which you can find security no matter what situation you are moving through in life. Examples include: creativity, resourcefulness, an appetite for learning, curiosity about the world, kindness, the ability to connect with people, playfulness, adaptability, being of service, goal aspiration, resilience, or a drive for self-improvement. No person and no circumstance can take any of these abilities away from you. You can be certain of that.

Week Four Checklist

You have been assigned four practices to work with this week.

- [ ] Practice examining your thoughts by writing them down and then challenging them using the questions provided earlier in the chapter.
- [ ] Explore judgment and compassion using the prompts provided. What do you gain from judging others? What stories do you tell yourself about what others think of you?
- [ ] Assess your own gut health using the questions provided, and add the three gut-healing foods (or an alternative that suits you) to your diet.
- [ ] Write down a list of qualities you know to be certain about yourself.

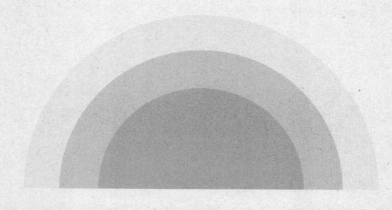

Week Five: A New Story

What Story Are You Telling Yourself?

As you now know, there's a story about your life that you tell yourself over and over in your subconscious mind. This story is the foundation of all the limiting belief systems that keep you feeling anxious, demotivated, and stuck. The story you tell about your past is what informs your expectations of your future. It casts a shadow of anticipated disappointment over what is to come for you. No wonder the future can seem so bleak.

Bridget came to me after experiencing a panic attack while driving home from work that knocked her off balance. She hadn't experienced anything like it for fifteen years while she was going about building a successful career in real estate with the ability to work whatever hours she wanted. She had a story about a painful childhood. Her parents divorced when she was two years old and, shortly after, her mother took her to Germany, far away from where her father lived. He never tried to contact her, never wrote a letter or visited. She grew up believing that her father had abandoned her and simply didn't care. Bridget was hesitant to explore her story—which is very common—as some parts made her feel sick with regret and shame. However, I knew that these painful emotions were exactly what we needed to dive into to release the heaviness she was carrying. As we worked through it together, she saw how the story of her life that she had been telling had led her to believe that men would always leave her; that she had to keep quiet and accept abusive behavior for fear of losing a man; and that after two failed marriages, there was no point in looking for love again. It simply felt too risky.

Bridget's past experiences with men had created a blueprint for her expectations of all other men in the future. She could not see an alternative because her mind was so fixed on telling the story this way. She felt hopeless, yearning for a love that was unavailable to her.

You have a story too, and it's an absolute gold mine—ready for you to dig out and break through those limiting beliefs that are holding you prisoner in a merry-go-round of high-functioning anxiety. The perfectionism, the pressure you place on yourself, the need to be busy all the time, the way you relate to people, and the way you speak to yourself all come back to the story you tell yourself about your life.

It's time to write out your story, unedited and true to your feelings. What story have you been telling about your life? Write out all that has gone wrong, all the key experiences that broke your heart or made you feel rejected, all the big moments when you were disappointed and hurt. It could be the story of a medical diagnosis, a partner who cheated, a parent's inconsistent love, a friend who turned on you, a painful divorce, a judgmental family member, a business that failed, the bullies at school, or the day you were fired from work. It's essential that you give yourself full permission to be the victim as you write this story. This is not the time to sugarcoat or find the silver lining. You will tell this story in this way for the very last time, so really take the opportunity to get it all out.

Take your time with it. It may feel exhausting and you will need to commit to the process, setting adequate time aside. But if you can work through this practice to completion, it is entirely worth it. You only need to do it once in your whole life. If you feel that you may need the support of a therapist, healer, or coach to guide you through the process, please do reach out for that support. Should the task feel too distressing for you, there is no need to force yourself. You can always come back to it at a later time when you feel ready.

Resist the urge to jump straight to the positive outlook, dismiss your feelings, or downplay your pain. It is important that you allow your pain and negative emotions to come up. You may feel the need to cry or get angry. Let this part of you have a voice. Welcome it in. Implement the tuning-in practice to work through your feelings without resistance and call on your loving parent as you need. The opportunity to rewrite your story is coming next.

Practice

Write out your life story as described here, breaking it down into a timeline to make it easier for yourself—like chapters of a book. Separate the chapters into increments of five years, starting with birth to five years old, six to ten years old, eleven to fifteen years old, and so on, all the way to the present. Fill in each chapter with dot points setting out the key moments. Then be sure to write about the way you felt, the meaning you made from each experience, and the beliefs you took on about yourself, about people, and about life. For each significant moment, ask yourself two questions: How did I feel? What did I make this mean?

When you are finished with the story, highlight all those core beliefs you've unearthed and write them out in a list so you can clearly see what you're working with. This process may require you to sit down for a few half-hour writing sessions over a number of days.

Rewrite Your Story

When Bridget had written out her old story and then rewritten it (which you'll do very soon), she found her heart bursting open with love. As she revisited memories from her childhood through her adult eyes, she awakened to the realization that her father had in fact loved her very much. He had tried to visit her multiple times and even wrote her letters, but her mother had kept it all hidden, as she was caught up in her bitterness toward him. She had only ever thought of herself. Bridget accessed a long-buried memory of her father standing in the front doorway of their house in Germany, pleading with her mother to let him see the children. He had done everything he could to keep his children in his life. Bridget was finally able to let in the love from her father that had been there all along. She could see that she was worthy of receiving it. She had always been worthy of love. This brought up a lot of anger toward her mother, which she was able to process. As she shed the heavy, limiting beliefs from the past and brought powerful awareness to them, Bridget felt open to new exciting possibilities for her future—including a fulfilling life with or without a partner. If a love worthy of her came her way, she was now ready to welcome it.

When you let go of your old story, you allow the Universe to write a new one for you. You open up to new possibilities as you liberate yourself from that unconscious, unaware telling of your life events. Writing your new story is about saying yes to your expansion and growth, and saying yes to the person you are becoming.

So how did Bridget rewrite her story? You will now be guided through this next step. First of all, make sure you've allowed some time to refresh between writing your old story and the new one. It may be enough to sleep on it or leave it for a few days, or you might like to go for a walk or make a cup of tea. Anything to create some space for your mind.

It is time to stop telling the old story now, to stop talking about the past in the way you have been. Unintentionally, we humans tend to lie about our past. Our story becomes embellished and dramatic as we cast meaning over the events with our creative, imaginative mind. Events that happened in your childhood become reasons why you are not good enough. To a child, life is confusing and the only way for children to make sense of what happens is to make it about them. "It's my fault," the child believes by default when they see their mother stressed or their father angry. This belief is keeping you anxious and feeding the fear. You can choose your story now.

Where did you tell yourself that what happened was your fault? Where did you blame yourself? Where have you believed you are not enough? Where did you think you were unloved, unwanted, or rejected, or that love was not available to you? These beliefs are all common in the developing mind, but they are not truth. They are all illusions that you are now going to challenge yourself to see through.

Can you see those events with more self-compassion, love, and forgiveness? You may need to forgive other people and you may need to forgive yourself. How can you give other people the benefit of the doubt? How can you take what happened less personally? Can you see the lovable, messy humanness in others' mistakes, and in your own? Can you see that the humans who upset you were doing their best—trying to survive, trying to be happy, trying to be liked, and trying to make it work with the resources, experiences, emotional intelligence, and spiritual growth available to them?

Can you see the lessons in what you went through? Can you feel grateful for what happened? Can you feel into a sense of awe for the wide scope of human experiences you've lived through on this wild, exhilarating roller-coaster ride of life?

Of course, in cases of abuse you are not required to forgive or feel grateful for what happened. You may like to reach out for the support of a therapist, healer, or coach to guide you through to a healing perspective.

If writing your story from a new perspective is feeling difficult for you to do, this is a very big sign that you are engaging in the most important and potentially rewarding healing work of your life. You have no choice but to grow. If you're feeling a lot of resistance, just notice how much you want to hang on to your old story and your pain. Get curious about it. What do you gain from believing that old story? If you're choosing to stay angry in blame and victimhood, you are holding on to a pain that only hurts you. Can you loosen your grip? Can you try to let go, to find peace? Can you imagine that there is another perspective available, even if you can't comprehend it yet, and acknowledge that you are in an illusion? Even this is a huge step forward to take.

Practice

Take a look at the old story of your life you have written out. Take a moment to thank this story for the role it has played in your life and the purpose it has served. Thank this story for getting you to where you are now.

Start to rewrite the big events in your life story that significantly affected you with a new perspective. Use the aforementioned guidance to choose the perspective that empowers you and helps you feel great about who you are and what you've lived through. This is the story of your life that you will tell going forward.

"Good and Bad" Doesn't Exist

Our experiences are neither good nor bad. They are neutral—until a human being comes along and gives the experience meaning. You might have learned that eating vegetables is good and eating fried food is bad. But what if the vegetables are presented to a two-year-old who dislikes bitter mush? What if the fried food is part of a celebration? You might believe a clean house is good and a messy house is bad. But what if maintaining constant cleanliness is a mental burden for you? What if allowing mess is a way for you to relax and practice letting go? Many of us think that death is bad and birth is good. But what if death is allowing someone who is in pain to find peace? Is it bad then? What if a birth results in significant trauma and injury for the mother? Is it still good? You might believe pain is bad and pleasure is good. But what if the pain is facilitating growth and a breakthrough? What if pleasure is keeping someone from dedicating themselves to a greater purpose in life?

Good cannot exist without bad and bad cannot exist without good. There is always duality in life. Both labels can exist together in the one circumstance. The beginning of a new relationship can feel like ecstasy, but as the years go on, the relationship will change. You may compare it to that initial phase, now long gone, and label the current version of the relationship bad. In some ways, all relationships must come to an end. The death of a loved one will be met with a sense of tragedy, but have you ever felt the stirring love emanating from the gathering of people at a funeral? Why is the ultimate value of a life defined by the fact that it ended? Isn't it a good thing that the life existed in the first place? If you think about the worst experiences you've been through and can extrapolate time far enough, you will find that some of the bad has transmuted into good somewhere along the line. No doubt your greatest challenges have contributed to the person you are today.

Similarly pain is nothing to fear or avoid. It is your greatest teacher. Without it, you wouldn't know the beauty of life's pleasures. There would be nothing to compare them to. A beautiful blue-sky day easily becomes boring when it is a daily occurrence. A blue sky after two weeks of rain, though, is something truly magical.

Life comes with neutral, interesting circumstances, one after the other, and it is your choice to label them good or bad or happy or sad. The meaning you make out of every experience is all yours.

Use this concept to finish rewriting your story and apply it to the parts where you feel stuck. What meaning do you want to make out of your life story? A triumphant, fulfilling, colorful, vibrant, and loving life story that serves you is entirely up to you. Choose that for yourself now.

Mental Notes

- The experiences of your life are neither good nor bad; they are neutral.
- You are the one choosing to apply the fixed label of good or bad to each experience.
- The meaning you make of your life events is entirely up to you. Why not choose to tell a life story that feels good to you?

Feeding Your Microbiome

The microbiome that lives in your gut is like a vibrant, life-giving garden, influencing the health of your body, mind, and brain. It is perhaps the most fascinating component of gut health that contributes to your Resilience Shield. A garden requires specific conditions to thrive, such as nutrients, water, and sunlight. Any change in these conditions can result in an overgrowth of weeds or the plants failing to thrive. Just as a beautiful garden can enhance your life, creating a beautiful gut garden is a powerful way to build your anxiety resilience.

You are inextricably linked to your microbiome. While half of you is made up of human cells, the other half is microorganism cells. It is estimated that the average person's microbiome contains 100 trillion microorganisms. These microorganisms include bacteria, yeasts, fungi, viruses, and protozoa, living together in harmony with you. This jungle of interdependent species lives within your gut, but also all over your skin, and in any mucous membranes such as the mouth, vagina, and lungs.

We will focus on the microbiome that lives predominantly within the gut, upon the lining of the intestines that you've been working to heal. The microbiome thrives in a healthy gut environment where the wall has been healed and soothed. In turn a healthy, balanced microbiome helps to protect the gut lining from inflammation. A balanced microbiome looks like a garden without many weeds, where the flowers flourish. Those flourishing flowers are the beneficial bacteria and microbes that can help raise the levels of calming chemicals in your brain, synthesize essential nutrients that you cannot otherwise make such as vitamin K and B vitamins, and produce soothing, anti-inflammatory short-chain fatty acids, all of which enhance your ability to cope with stress and reduce anxiety.

The picture is a little different in most of our gut gardens, thanks again to modern life. Usually we have some harmful, pathogenic species of bacteria or other microbes living within us. Even beneficial species can overgrow, causing problems. Think of this like your flower bed growing out from its parameters, forming unsightly, uneven patches all over the lawn. An imbalance of the gut microbiome can release harmful lipopolysaccharides—chemicals that promote inflammation, damaging the gut lining—as well as crowd out the good guys, taking up residence in their homes.

Fiber and Prebiotics

In order to balance the microbiome, you must provide your beneficial microbes all their favorite foods, so that they have plenty to eat. Your good bacteria absolutely love to eat an abundance of fiber, prebiotics, and polyphenols. Prebiotics are a specific type of fiber that are even more powerful for increasing populations of beneficial bacteria and directly help digestive symptoms such as diarrhea and constipation. Increasing your fiber intake overall helps maintain regular bowel movements, balance blood sugar, and keep you full.

Women typically require about 25 grams of fiber each day, whereas men require 30 grams. To include more fiber in your day, try to leave the skin on the vegetables and fruit you eat and choose smoothies over juices (the juicing process usually results in fiber being removed). Be sure to include chickpeas, beans, lentils, oats, quinoa, chia seeds, and pepitas in your diet, with green vegetables such as broccoli, spinach, and kale.

Being mindful of your refined sugar intake from foods such as lollipops, potato chips, white bread, and cookies and replacing them with more high-fiber fruits, vegetables, nuts, seeds, and whole grains will help shift the microbiome balance to a higher population of beneficial bacteria.

Here is a list with examples of the grams of fiber per serving found in different foods, so you can ensure you're getting enough each day:

- 1 apple = 4.4 grams
- 1 cup black beans = 15 grams
- 1 cup cooked brown rice = 3.5 grams (compared to just 0.4 grams found in 1 cup of white rice)
- 1 cup cooked oats = 4 grams
- 1 cup lentils = 16 grams
- 1 cup sweet potato = 4 grams
- 1 handful pepitas = 5 grams

I also recommend adding some key prebiotic foods into your regular diet, as per your tolerance. Here are some that your good gut bacteria especially love to eat:

- apples
- asparagus
- banana (green, underripe)
- chicory root
- dandelion greens
- flaxseeds
- garlic
- Jerusalem artichoke
- konjac root
- leeks
- oats
- onions
- raw cacao

It is quite common to experience more gas and bloating as you increase your intake of fiber and prebiotic-rich foods, particularly if you get very enthusiastic about it. This will be temporary, usually lasting no more than twenty-four hours. My advice is to go slow, adding an extra heaped tablespoon serving of these foods per meal at a time, and build your way up to eating more and more of these foods. If you experience gas, you've gone a little too far, so pull back. Over time, you will tolerate a higher intake of high-fiber and prebiotic foods, and this is the goal.

Polyphenols

Healthy gut microbes also love to eat polyphenols, which are found in the natural color pigment in fruits and vegetables. This is where the common advice to "eat the rainbow" truly applies. Polyphenols increase the diversity and population of good bacteria such as Lactobacillus and Bifidobacteria while also reducing the growth of pathogenic microbes. Polyphenols provide an antioxidant action, which protects cells from pathogen damage. Their unique chemical structure activates beneficial bacterial activity and switches off the activity of harmful pathogenic bacteria. In doing so, they have an overall regulatory effect that balances the microbiome. If in doubt, just add some extra color onto your plate every day.

Here is a list of foods that are great sources of polyphenols to inspire you:

- almonds, hazelnuts, pecans
- apricots, pears, plums
- beetroot
- blackberries, blueberries, raspberries, strawberries
- black or green tea, coffee (caffeine-free green tea is best; be sure to limit your caffeine intake, as per your tolerance)

- broccoli
- dark chocolate, raw cacao
- kale, spinach
- olives
- red wine (one standard glass)

Probiotics and Fermented Foods

Probiotic, fermented foods such as tempeh, kefir, natural unsweetened yogurt, sourdough, kimchi, sauerkraut, and kombucha are also helpful, as they encourage and support a healthy gut environment.

Whether in the form of capsules or foods, probiotics do not colonize the gut microbiome with beneficial bacteria species as we once thought. However, they do exert an overall anti-inflammatory effect that encourages your existing microbiome to flourish. Probiotics will also help to reduce symptoms such as diarrhea, loose stools, and constipation, which people with anxiety commonly experience. If you're wondering whether to take a daily probiotic capsule or not, it can certainly have a positive impact, but the effect will only last for as long as you're taking the capsules. The most important thing to keep in mind over the long term is feeding your gut microbiome the prebiotic foods it thrives on in the first place.

Here are some probiotic foods that you can include in your daily diet:

- kefir
- kimchi
- kombucha
- sauerkraut
- sourdough bread

- tempeh (fermented soy)
- yogurt (natural, unsweetened)

Practice

Add in more fiber, prebiotic foods, fermented/probiotic foods, and polyphenols into your diet, as per the guidelines in this section. Measuring exact quantities is less important than simply making an effort to consume more of these foods and keeping them at the top of your mind.

Remember that it is normal to experience a little more gas as you add these foods in and your body adjusts, because the gut microbes literally ferment these foods into gas as they eat them. If you feel particularly uncomfortable, pull back on your intake and slowly build up a little more each day.

If you suffer from painful bloating and general digestive discomfort, always consult your healthcare practitioner to ensure that this is the right advice to follow for your individual situation. In these cases, often a much slower, gentler approach is required as these foods are introduced.

Week Five Checklist

For Week Five you have three practices to complete—including the significant task of writing and rewriting your story. It is normal for this task to take longer than one week to complete.

- ☐ Write out your old life story, breaking it down into chapters of key events.
- ☐ Review your old story, thanking it for the role it has played in your life, and then rewrite it—creating a new empowered and helpful story to tell from here on.
- ☐ Add in more fiber, prebiotic foods, fermented/probiotic foods, and polyphenols into your diet, as per the guidelines suggested.

Week Six: Making Miracles

Acts of Service

When you're struggling with your inner world, you naturally focus on yourself. You think about how you look, instead of how you can make another person feel with your smile and your listening ears. You worry about what you're doing with your life, instead of doing something helpful for someone else with the power and resources you already have. You tell a story that you aren't a worthy person, instead of using your two valuable hands to help out a friend by preparing food or massaging their aching shoulders—an act of service they would truly treasure. You fixate on what isn't enough in you and all your brokenness and forget all about the power you have to make a valuable, positive impact on the world.

While it is important to receive love and support from others and not move purely into a state of giving to others and being of service, there is one surefire way to turn a downward mental health spiral around. Ask yourself: What is one thing I can do today to make somebody else's life a little easier?

As you shift your focus to what you can do and what value you can offer to another human being, you automatically feel more valuable in yourself. You feel the heartwarming sense of making a contribution to the world that, in your own small way, actually makes it a better place. With one simple approach you are meeting three of your basic mental health needs: connection and belonging, self-worth and significance, and purpose and contribution.

> ## Practice
>
> You may already be a generous, thoughtful human being, but this week you're going to make even more of a conscious effort to serve. Take a moment to consider the people around you. Who needs help in some area? Where could you assist?
>
> Examples to inspire you in this task might include: preparing a meal for someone; writing a letter of appreciation to a friend who has been there for you; cleaning someone's house or car; repairing something broken for another person; sending a thoughtful message to check in with a colleague; leaving a note for someone that brings them a smile; offering a hug; and holding space as someone else speaks their mind, uninterrupted.

Making Miracles

For how long have you been moving blindly through the motions of your daily life, deep in your own worries and insecurities? When your focus is internal, your world can feel tiny, like it could all fit into the four walls of the room you are in. It is no wonder this closed state of anxiety has you feeling limited, stuck, and fearful.

I lived this way for years after my parents' divorce: head down, blinders on. I'd wake up and robotically stare at my phone. The peace of my slumber quickly dissipated as I scrolled through filtered images of the better lives everyone else was living. I felt numb as I consumed a horrific news story or was jolted by the violent remembering of my long to-do list. I felt as though something was chasing me, but I couldn't have told you what it was. My anxious mind would creep in, clawing on my consciousness, spewing out a story of how stressful, unpleasurable, and bleak my day ahead would be. That there was no magic coming my way. My best days were behind me anyway, it told me. The joy was lost in those faded memories of first-kiss butterflies; playing in make-believe houses; the limitlessness of my first time driving a car alone; travels to hot, exotic places; falling dizzily in love. I already knew how good life could get and it was all downhill from here. My remaining years would be mediocre at best. Yet my brain still craved hits of dopamine—those moments of magic. It sought pleasure in bingeing on decadent foods; buying new clothes; dreaming of how perfect I could be if I just got fitter and healthier; and hitting my next assignment submission date, leading to an obsessive study routine. It's safe to say I was looking in all the wrong places for little miracles to take me away from my mundane life. Something wasn't working.

So I began to ponder. What if I could create meaningful miracles in my daily life, in a functional and sustainable way? Could that even be possible? What if I could feel alive without needing to jump on a plane, or out of one, or kill myself working all year just to spend one week in a five-star resort? What if I could feel like I was truly living an engaged, fulfilled life anywhere, at any time? As I asked these questions I started to realize I had power within me to control my outlook—and you have it too. We all have the power to perceive our lives in a way that feels miraculous, alive, and wonderful. We can take off the blinders of fear and choose to open our perception with love. This is how we make miracles.

American playwright Thornton Wilder once said, "We can only be said to be truly alive in those moments when our hearts are conscious of our treasures." What everyone seeks in those big moments in life—in otherworldly travel, momentous celebrations, stunning natural landscapes, the birth of a new human, career achievements, and falling in love—are moments of exhilarating awe and wonder. Moments where your heart is wide open, where you can't believe they said "Yes!" or that life could be so incredibly beautiful. Moments where it feels good to be alive.

The examples here are the miracles of life that are impossible to ignore. They're big, loud, and obvious. They may feel all too rare, or expensive and out of reach. But these examples are not all there is. There are miracles unfolding around you that you ignore without meaning to, simply because you're focused on yourself and your problems. The flow of life around you—with its infinite complexities, profound beauty, and unexpected synchronicities—is a miracle you no doubt shut yourself off from. How many miracles are trying to find you?

When I picture myself years ago, waking up and reaching for my phone to be sucked into my inner turmoil, I wonder what miracles I didn't see. What if I'd noticed the glint of sunlight pouring in through the windows? What if I'd noticed that my body had kept me breathing all night, without my input, somehow working automatically for me? What if I'd considered how wonderfully soft and comfortable my bed felt beneath me? What if I'd appreciated how good my hair smelled, because I had access to a shower and nice-smelling shampoo? What if I'd found pleasure in knowing I had a kitchen full of food—delicious, quality food I had chosen because I had that luxury? What if I'd tried to count the thousand possible ways I could enjoy myself that day? What if I'd thought about all the good that happens in this world—the smiles, the hugs, and the love expressed between humans, and the gorgeous fact that we're put on this planet to love one another? What if I'd looked out the window at the spectacular shapes and colors of the trees, or the interesting, funny characters walking down the street? What if I'd asked myself what I could see that was going *right* today and working well for me? What if I'd smiled with satisfaction at my good health and access to top-quality medical care, should I ever need it? What if I'd considered how fortunate I was to be born in a country with such freedom and opportunity? What if I'd questioned even the chances and serendipitous moments that had to occur for me to be born and be alive in this moment? Just so you know, the chance of being born is estimated at one in 400 quadrillion to ten to the 2.64 millionth power. In other words, the chances are so low that your brain can't even numerically process what kind of magic took place to make you. What if I'd taken a few seconds to consider that my life, my plain existence, my being here in this moment right now, was a miracle?

Now you may be wondering what it is that you're missing. There are always miracles around you. Can you see them? Can you actively channel your power of perception into love, and look for them? When you look for miracles, more will appear. Come back to remembering that your life is a miracle too.

Mental Notes

- You can make miracles happen in your daily life if you activate them with your focus.
- Remember that your very existence is a miracle all on its own.

Practice

Every day this week, write out an entire page in your journal noting the miracles around you. Express gratitude for all the stunning intricacies and mind-boggling complexities and synchronicities of life around you. You'll notice that, as the ball gets rolling, this process becomes easier and flows out of you without the same effort it takes to begin. Be patient with yourself and curious about all the miracles you haven't noticed. Start noticing.

Nutrition Myths

I had been alive for almost twenty-one years when I first truly understood that the food I ate at every meal was an opportunity to nourish my body. I took my place in a healthy cooking class in the Byron Bay hinterland, seated at a table covered in bunches of homegrown bananas, labeled glass jars of colorful spices, macadamia nuts, roasted pumpkin halves, and bowls of bitter greens and edible yellow flower petals. It clicked. Every bite I ate was adding to nutrient stores in my cells that could have an impact on my overall well-being. I was led through a rustic kitchen garden, where I was introduced to herbs that could cure a toothache, soothe itchy skin, or help relieve depression. Finally the dots connected between what grew from the ground and my own body.

For twenty-one years I'd seen food as simply a means to cure my hunger and, later, as something to restrict and fight against. My hunger was inconvenient and my food intake felt like a battle to control. It was a daily source of anxious turmoil. "Am I eating too much? How can I distract myself so I will skip a meal? I shouldn't be eating this. I should be good. I should be better. Oh, screw it. It's all too hard. I'll just give in. Now I feel horrible about myself...." And so the cycle went on.

I set out to learn everything I could about the components of the food I ate. Seeing food as the foundation for a great mood, energy, strong fingernails, and healthy hair helped a lot on the days when my anxious mind tempted me not to eat. Nutrition is a key component of the Resilience Shield.

Studying nutrition for four years, I went through waves of extreme opinion on certain topics. From the never-good-enough vegan to the weight-loss-disguised-as-keto and paleo diets, to obsessive-compulsive clean eating and organic puritanism, to the vilification of soy and gluten. I always thought at least I couldn't go wrong with fruits and vegetables, but soon I discovered even those had issues. Beetroot and spinach were denied for a time due to the potentially harmful lectins, as well as phytates and oxalates, which are said to block mineral absorption. Consuming too much kale was considered potentially dangerous for the thyroid.

It was getting ridiculous. I was running out of foods I could eat. My determination to get it perfect was only increasing my anxiety. So I stepped back and took a good look at myself, viewing all the rabbit holes I'd been down from a distance.

When you're making arguments against a wholesome vegetable, you know you've definitely gone too deep into the craziness of the nutrition world. A nutrition lecturer helped validate my dawning conclusion—that there's a strong argument for and against almost every food or diet. No matter what you do, it could be argued that it is no good. My food perfectionism finally gave way to a much more relaxed approach combining intuition, knowledge, and common sense.

Clients will often share with me fifteen-second videos or bite-size information posts about the harmful effects of one nutrient, diet, or food, or lists of foods that increase anxiety, in fear that they need to stop consuming them. It is important to keep in mind that a social media platform is a marketing platform. To market and sell, these platforms must grab attention. Content that shocks or sits on either side of the extremes of nutrition will always grab attention and help sell. We must also remember the importance of quality research and context, as one sentence on Instagram taken out of the context of a complex discussion can easily create alarm. For example, yes, if you consume too much kale you could theoretically disrupt the function of your thyroid gland. However, the amount required for that problem to occur is far greater than anyone would ever consume (we're talking bucketloads), so the real-life concern is unnecessary. Let's take a look at some of these so-called dangerous ingredients and diets through an informed and practical lens.

Gluten

A gluten-free diet may not reduce anxiety, even in those who have Celiac disease, which requires an official diagnosis with your health-care practitioner.[1] A gluten-free diet may be beneficial if you notice a difference and are genuinely gluten-sensitive, which can be confirmed through a HLA-DQ gene test. However, removing gluten-containing foods from the diet results in a reduction of microbiome diversity, meaning less life flourishing in your gut garden.[2] If you do not notice a difference whether you eat gluten or not, you should not exclude it altogether from your food intake and it is unlikely to make any difference to anxiety. Besides, sourdough toast makes Sunday brunch a whole lot more delicious.

Sugar

A sugar-free diet is unlikely to make a significant difference to anxiety for most people. The research is conflicting and inconsistent, and it is very difficult to determine causality between sugar intake and anxiety.[3] That's because there are so many factors involved in anxiety, as you now know. So you can rest assured that a bit of chocolate after dinner or an ice cream in summer can remain in your life. Remember that sugar resides in many foods we eat, including fruit, carrots, beetroot, bread, and pasta, not just sweets. Sugar is just energy for your body. Some sugars come with more nutrients and some come with less. A sudden large intake of sugar can, however, create temporary havoc with your blood sugar levels, which is not the best thing for anxiety. This is not such a problem if sugary foods are consumed alongside a source of protein, fat, and fiber, and form part of a balanced diet. You will learn precisely how to do that later in this chapter.

Dairy

There is no clear association between the consumption of dairy and anxiety.[4] Some studies suggest that including dairy has benefits, and many dairy products form the basis of probiotic, fermented foods, such as kefir and yogurt. The Mediterranean diet is heralded as one of the most evidence-based health-promoting diets in the world, particularly for improving mental health, and it includes dairy products.[5]

Animal Products

It is true that adding more plants to your diet is a good thing for your mental health resilience overall. Nuts, seeds, vegetables, and fruits are nutrient-dense foods that support human health in a myriad of ways, from increasing the diversity of the gut microbiome to reducing inflammation. The strict exclusion of animal products is not necessary to achieve these benefits. In fact, a critical review demonstrated that in eleven of the eighteen studies referenced, with research gathered from more than 160,000 individuals across the world, there was poorer psychological health in those who abstained entirely from meat and seafood consumption.[6] The benefits, especially for people with high-functioning anxiety, may be less about removing meat and more about adding in more colorful, fresh vegetables.

When it comes to mastering your anxious mind, you're much better off having the least amount of restriction around eating as possible, allowing for the opportunity to connect to your body's signals and intuitive impulses to guide you. The aim is not to have a perfect diet. The aim is to nourish your body so you feel calm and relaxed. Look for the forest, not the trees. Unless you have specific health goals and you're working with a trained professional dietician or nutritionist, forget the messy, confusing, inconsistent nitty-gritty details. One thing the research seems to agree on is the positive impact of a nutritious, minimally processed diet for mental health.[7] Aim for a more nutrient-dense diet more of the time with room for flexibility and be sure to embrace eating as one of life's great joys.

Practice

Can you avoid the labels good *and* bad when it comes to food?

Can you allow for balance, fewer rules, and more flexibility in your eating habits?

The Macronutrients

The macronutrients are the three components that make up every food we consume: protein, carbohydrates, and fats. Each macronutrient is important for building anxiety resilience in different ways, and I recommend that you include a balance of each macronutrient on your plate. Think of this part like learning a language or the poses in yoga. Once you are familiar with the basic principles, you can flow fluently with the information as you make your food choices.

Protein

The main sources of protein include eggs, meat, fish, nuts, seeds, legumes, and dairy products. Protein is an essential dietary requirement every single day. It forms the building blocks of your entire body, and it is important for maintaining healthy skin, hair, nails, and lining of your gut. Your body requires the amino acids that make up protein to make serotonin, GABA, and other calming, happy-brain chemicals that support your mental health. Protein promotes muscle growth, regulates the digestive process, keeps you feeling full between meals, and stabilizes your blood sugar.

Blood sugar regulation is essential for improving anxiety resilience, as a sudden spike and drop in the level will lead to anxiety. I always feel anxious if I leave too much time between meals, especially if I forget to eat lunch. Within a few minutes of eating, I feel calm again and can think clearly. There's a reason we get "hangry" and irritable if we don't eat when we need to.

Aim for a serving of protein with every meal. A main-meal serving size of protein could be two eggs; a can of tuna; a palm-size portion of salmon, chicken, or tempeh; or a palm-size mix of lentils, chickpeas, beans, quinoa, nuts, and seeds. Protein powders are another easy way to boost your intake.

Most women require between 40 to 60 grams of protein daily while men need around 60 to 80 grams per day. Keep in mind that activity levels also contribute to your individual daily protein requirements; the more activity you do, the more protein you should eat.

Carbohydrates

Complex carbohydrates are found in fruits, vegetables, grains (including oats and rice), and wholegrain pasta. Simple carbohydrates are refined, processed foods such as baked goods. Carbohydrates provide energy to the brain, keep your periods regular, help you ovulate, support your metabolism, reduce premenstrual syndrome (PMS) symptoms, and keep your mood balanced and energy level stable. Complex carbohydrates contain antioxidants and fiber that support a healthy microbiome and cells.

Carbohydrates tell your brain that you're safe. There's no famine going on and there's plenty of food available. When your intake of carbohydrates is too low, your level of stress hormone cortisol rises. An adequate intake of carbohydrates reduces stress and calms your body.

It's particularly important to listen to your body when it comes to carbohydrates. I recommend adding some in with every meal and avoiding counting or measuring your intake unless advised by a healthcare practitioner.

Fats

Fats include avocado, olive oil, coconut products, nuts, seeds, and oily fish such as salmon, sardines, and tuna. Every cell in your body is protected by a cell membrane made of fat. Your hormones are created using fat, so a healthy fat intake will help keep your hormones in balance. Fats combined with carbohydrates and protein will help slow the release of sugar into your bloodstream, keeping your blood sugar levels stable. Every cell in your brain is protected by a fatty myelin sheath, and healthy fats can help reduce inflammation. A brain with less inflammation is better able to balance out the brain chemicals that stabilize your mood and keep you feeling calm.

Aim to add one tablespoon or a two-finger-size portion of healthy fats to every meal.

Building a Calm Plate

The process of putting together a nutritious meal can be overwhelming for many people—particularly if you're experiencing anxiety. But when you break it down and simplify the process, you'll find it is easy to apply. In this section you will find the five principle steps I follow as I put a meal together. This approach is far better for your consistency long term than following a series of recipes. This way, you can choose the foods you enjoy and are already familiar with to create endless combinations of nourishing buddha bowls, salads, stir-fries, and other delicious meals. Just add some tasty spices, such as turmeric, paprika, cumin, cinnamon, chili, garlic, and garden herbs, experimenting with the flavors you like, and you will be cooking like a naturopath in no time.

Step One: Where Is the Protein?

Include a palm-size serving with each meal. Options include:

- **Animal protein:** chicken, eggs, feta, fish (especially mackerel, salmon, sardines, and tuna), grass-fed beef, goat cheese, halloumi, lamb, natural yogurt, seafood (oysters, prawns, and scallops), and turkey
- **Nuts and seeds:** almonds, Brazil nuts, chia seeds, hemp seeds, peanuts, pecans, pistachios, pumpkin seeds, sunflower seeds, and walnuts
- **Plant protein:** black beans, buckwheat, cannellini beans, chickpeas (drained and rinsed), edamame beans, fermented organic soy, fermented rice or pea protein powder (such as Amazonia Raw Vanilla), lentils, mushrooms, quinoa, and tempeh

Step Two: Choose Your Vegetables

Include a one cup serving with each meal. Options include:

- **Bitter greens:** chicory, nasturtium leaves, parsley, rocket
- **Complex carbohydrates:** beetroot, carrot, fennel, parsnip, potato, pumpkin, sweet potato, and turnip
- **Cruciferous vegetables:** broccoli, brussels sprouts, cabbage, cauliflower, and kale
- **Dark leafy greens:** bok choy, broccoli, broccolini, chard, kale, and spinach
- **High polyphenols (color) and prebiotic fiber:** all dark leafy greens, artichoke, asparagus, beetroot, bell peppers or capsicum, carrot, celery, garlic, lettuce, olives, onion, pumpkin, radishes, shallots, sweet potato, tomato, and watercress

Step Three: Add Your Fats

Try to have one tablespoon or a two-finger-size serving with each meal. Fats feed your brain and hormones. Options include:

- Avocado, coconut cream, coconut flakes, coconut oil, fresh coconut, flaxseed oil, olive oil, and olives
- **Fatty fish:** mackerel, sardines, salmon, and tuna
- **Nuts and seeds:** almonds, Brazil nuts, chia seeds, flaxseeds, hemp seeds, pecans, pistachios, pumpkin seeds, sunflower seeds, and walnuts

Try to have at least two servings of fatty fish per week.

Step Four: Is There Enough Fiber and Color?

Include one serving with each meal. Options include:

- Cocoa, dark chocolate, green tea, and spices
- **High polyphenols (color):** all dark leafy greens, beetroot, bell peppers or capsicum, black beans, blackberries, blueberries, carrot, lettuce, olives, pineapple, pumpkin, radishes, raspberries, red onion, shallots, spices (chili, cinnamon, cumin, paprika, turmeric), spinach, strawberries, sweet potato, tomato, and watercress
- **High prebiotic fiber:** almonds, apples, apricots, artichoke, asparagus, beans, brown rice, chickpeas, chicory root, dandelion greens, dates, figs, garlic, green bananas, hazelnuts, Jerusalem onion, leek, lentils, nuts and seeds, oats, pawpaw, pears, pecans, plums, and prunes

Leave the skin on fruit and vegetables for extra fiber and choose smoothies over juices.

Step Five: Do You Have Plenty of Carbohydrates?

Include one serving with each meal. Options include:

- **Fruit:** apricots, bananas, blueberries, dates, figs, mango, pawpaw, peaches, pineapple, prunes, raspberries, and strawberries
- **Vegetables:** beetroot, carrot, potato, pumpkin, and sweet potato
- **Whole grains:** amaranth, beans, black rice, brown rice, buckwheat, corn, legumes, lupin, millet, oats, polenta, quinoa, red rice, rye, sourdough bread, and spelt

Practice

Consider the macronutrients on your plate as you prepare or choose your meals. Follow the five steps discussed to build a calm plate, balanced with all the protein, carbohydrates, and fats you need.

Week Six Checklist

In Week Six I've given you four practices to work with. You may find these tasks a little less time-consuming, so you'll have space to complete the exercise of rewriting your story if need be.

☐ Make a more conscious effort to serve. Consider the people around you who may need your help this week.

☐ Write out an entire page in your journal each day noting the miracles around you.

☐ Avoid labeling foods good and bad, and consider how you might reduce the rules you have around food if your eating has been rigid.

☐ Apply what you have learned about building a calm plate.

Week Seven: Pleasure

The Art of Pleasure

Daniella had just been promoted to a new role at work that would demand more of her time. It was a big step up in her career and something she had been working toward for years. This was a dream come true, and yet she was freaking out. Already her week was packed with running a house, managing a renovation, trying to fit in Pilates classes, and taking care of her young son. Her partner was equally time poor, busy running his business. When she came to see me, Daniella was overwhelmed by her life and terrified that her partner would leave her. They had completely lost their spark, she told me. They had barely touched each other in weeks and every day they were arguing. I encouraged Daniella to listen to what her fear was trying to tell her. As we explored this fear openly, it became clear how much Daniella had lost the spark within *herself*. She was on her way to burnout and disconnected from her body and her feminine energy state.

Every human being, regardless of gender, can embody either feminine or masculine energy. Each person usually feels more at home in one state over the other, but we actually need a balance between the two. High-functioning anxiety will drive many people too far into their masculine state of *doing*: working endlessly and taking on the burdens of life on their own. There is nothing wrong with this when it is balanced with gentle, restorative feminine energy. However, the masculine energy of productivity is far more celebrated in society than the feminine, which is shamed as lazy and indulgent. So the feminine way is neglected while the masculine is prioritized. It is no wonder that anxiety comes along, reminding us we've fallen way out of alignment with the feminine state.

While Daniella was operating well in her masculine energy, and being rewarded with results in her career and the promise of a beautiful renovated house, deep down she was yearning to be in her slower, more receptive feminine state. If you're reading this book, whatever gender you identify with, no doubt you feel this yearning to connect more strongly with the feminine energy of being.

Bringing her masculine energy home day after day, Daniella was finding that the dynamic with her partner was neutralizing to a masculine–masculine energy. For attraction to occur in any kind of romantic relationship there needs to be a positive and a negative charge, like two opposing ends of a magnet. In this situation, Daniella was expressing more frustration toward her partner than love. Her partner, in turn, was treating her more as a business associate than a lover. Her work was to reconnect with her feminine energy, including her body and senses. It was about actively inviting in pleasure.

Daniella began by dancing for five minutes every morning to whatever music inspired her to move. Within just a few days, she noticed she felt softer with herself and more open toward her partner. They began to reconnect. She also told me that the practice helped work feel more manageable. This simple ritual gave her the space she needed to feel into her heart and replenish herself in the feminine state, so she could be more effective in the masculine *doing* energy— and, more importantly, feel balanced within.

When your heart is filled with creativity, love, slowness, joy, and pleasure, so much in life falls back into place. It may seem backward, but it is from this state that clarity, inspired ideas, and solutions come. This is where you'll find true control when life feels out of control. Slow down. Stop. Connect back with your heart, your body, and what makes you feel alive. Could anxiety be the warning signal that your heart is draining dry of passion? An activated nervous system riddled with anxiety will send you further into rigidity, plan-setting, worry, endless rumination, and tension in the body. Your work is to become conscious of the pattern and change direction. Moving toward pleasure is one pathway you can travel to get back into alignment with your feminine energy.

When you are in a state of fear and anxiety, your awareness is very much centered in the mind—up high around your head somewhere. You're disconnected from your body, from your senses, from the present moment, and far off in some abstract thought about something irrelevant to the experience of being alive right now. Have you ever had a massage and noticed that you weren't really there for it? Only during the last half hour did you really relax and feel your mind wind down. Have you ever wolfed down your lunch so you could continue typing an email, not even noticing the taste? Have you ever lived an entire day in your incredible, alive human body, and not really felt anything much? (Except anxiety.) This is why it is so easy to forget to eat, or eat beyond satiation, when you're anxious. Being up in your head means you can push yourself beyond your limits and your body's signals. It's how you learned to cope with a busy, challenging life and a world that glorifies constant *doing*. When you draw your focus and awareness down into your body, you naturally feel more connected and grounded.

Pleasure is about so much more than the realms of sexuality, as people often assume when they see this word. Pleasure can be anything that delights your senses of sight, taste, smell, touch, and sound. It's about shifting into your slower, more open, and receptive feminine energy—letting go of the race, the shoulds, and the imaginary deadlines. Giving yourself permission to truly feel life's pleasures becomes easier when you understand the power in this practice. See, real control comes from a slower pace: where the mind has the space and time to access deep wisdom, innovation, and inspiration to solve the problems you face. When you force and struggle your way through daily life, there is no space for the ideas that truly catapult you forward.

Practicing the art of pleasure could mean spending time at the beach, actively tuning in to the feeling of the sun on your skin, appreciating the scent of salt in the air, and marveling at the spectacle of bright blue ocean waves crashing before your eyes. It could be curiously tracing the soft edge of a bright pink flower. It could mean being fully present as you inhale the layers of complexity from the lotion you apply to your hands. It might be slowly sipping your cup of tea, noticing the way the fragrant liquid slides down your throat and warms your belly. It could be moving your limbs and hips to the rhythm of your favorite music, without a care for how you look—simply enjoying the freedom of intuition-led movement.

You may think you surround yourself with pleasures already: delicious food, scented candles, baths, artwork, music, soft clothing, and so on. But there is a big difference between being present and actively engaged in the experience and simply moving through the motions so you can tick off some self-care. Anxiety will have you tuning out the pleasures available to you. If you're zoned out and lost in rumination, you miss so many of the gifts that life is bringing to you. The cycle strengthens as you reinforce anxiety-inducing beliefs, such as believing there's not enough magic here for you. You can make almost any simple moment extraordinarily pleasurable if you engage your senses. Taking a shower can just be taking a shower, or it can be a feast for the senses: noticing the temperature, the pressure, the sensation of water trickling down your skin, and the scents of the products you use. The key is remembering to look out for the pleasures that are available, activating your senses, and being present with the experience.

Mental Notes

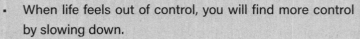

- When life feels out of control, you will find more control by slowing down.
- Focus on what brings pleasure to your senses, brings you out of your mind and down into your body, where you can literally feel grounded.

Practice

This week, practice the art of pleasure. Create space in your day just for you to experience pleasure, and weave moments of pleasure into your day. Play music. Dance with free movement. Taste your food. Appreciate the scents around you. Enjoy a longer shower than usual. Wear clothing that feels good. Take care of your skin. Massage your own neck, hands, or feet. Simply ask yourself: How can I invite in more pleasure?

Knowing Your Hormone Cycle

Nicola was about to get married. She was a wedding planner herself, so to be finally planning her own wedding was something she'd been dreaming about for years. And yet she couldn't understand why some weeks she felt on top of the world and other weeks she'd fall flat into a mess of sadness, self-doubt, and anxiety. She berated herself for never being consistently motivated to complete her daily tasks or stick to her workout goals in the lead-up to the wedding. When she came to me, she was deep into another anxiety episode and desperate for help to ensure her day wouldn't be ruined by these intense feelings. I asked her if she was tracking her monthly cycle. She looked back at me, eyes wide like this was a test and she had failed. I could tell that her hormone cycle was impacting her anxiety. Here was a woman driving a car blind. So it is to live life as a menstruating woman, not knowing your hormone cycle.

Hormonal balance is the next key element of the Resilience Shield we will explore. If you are a woman, or assigned female at birth, you are not the same person every day. You have different energy levels, social tendencies, working capacity, and needs depending on the phase of your menstrual cycle you're in. There are four key phases to the cycle, and I like to think of them in terms of seasons: menstruation (winter), follicular phase (spring), ovulation (summer), and luteal phase (autumn). Knowing these phases means you can be a whole lot kinder to yourself when you're not at peak productivity, and make the most of your surges of motivation and inspiration when you have them. If you can start to align your life to your cycles, you can flow gracefully and peacefully with the natural rhythms within you.

Menstruation (Winter)

It begins with your period, the first day of which is day one of your cycle—your inner winter. Estrogen and progesterone levels drop to allow the shedding of the endometrial lining. Your energy levels may be lower during your days of heaviest bleeding, and you might naturally prefer spending more time in your own company. You'll experience heightened creativity, so this is a good time to generate new ideas and set new intentions. Make plans for the month ahead and be extra gentle with yourself. You might like to meditate, take warm baths, spend time in nature, and enjoy low-intensity physical activity such as yoga or walking.

Bleeding should last three to seven days, with only mild if any cramping pain. Nausea and debilitating pain is not normal and should be investigated with your healthcare practitioner. Temporary digestive symptoms such as bloating and loose stools can occur.

Follicular Phase (Spring)

Following on from menstruation is your inner springtime. Estrogen levels start to rise, thickening the endometrial lining, and cervical fluid is produced. You can always count on your energy levels and motivation returning at this time, even if your luteal phase had you fearing they were gone forever. You'll naturally want to reach out to friends and socialize while feeling more motivated to act on your goals and say yes to more projects. Now is the time to execute your plans, work out more intensely, use the heightened motivation to your advantage, explore new things, and enjoy others' company.

Ovulation (Summer)

Ovulation is your inner summer and always occurs ten to fourteen days before your next period. This is the menstrual cycle's main event. Variations in your ovulation day can easily occur and the best way to know is to track your fertility signs, including cervical fluid and charting your temperature. Your energy levels will be peaking, you'll feel confident, you will likely notice your libido rising, and you'll naturally enjoy being social and taking action. Your estrogen levels are soaring, with follicle-stimulating hormone and luteinizing hormone to allow for the egg to release into the fallopian tubes, where it will remain alive for just twenty-four hours unless it is fertilized. The unfertilized egg cell forms an entire gland called the corpus luteum, which releases progesterone—one of the most important female reproductive hormones. Understanding progesterone is essential for building your anxiety resilience. You can only make progesterone through ovulation.

Luteal Phase (Autumn)

The luteal phase is your inner autumn, where progesterone rises and signifies that ovulation has occurred. This phase usually lasts for ten to fourteen days. It's time to slow down, take on less work, and turn inward to your emotional world. This is where many women will experience PMS symptoms including anxiety.

What Is Premenstrual Syndrome?

You may already be familiar with feeling a clockwork drop in your mood and rise in fatigue and anxiety each month before your period. This is the time most women will feel more sensitive and irritable, less motivated to work, and perhaps sad for no reason. It is usual for the emotions you've suppressed through the ups and downs of the month to surface at this time, ready for release. This is a wonderful built-in emotional recharge system that clears out any murkiness you may be holding on to, readying you for a new month. It's like a wave at the ocean shoreline, the ebb before the flow. For most women, the invitation is to simply allow the slowing-down process and accept that it can be normal for your Resilience Shield to be affected by the natural fluctuations of your hormone cycle. There isn't necessarily anything wrong with you or your hormones if you feel drawn into your inner world in the days before you bleed.

PMS is a combination of different symptoms such as anxiety, anger outbursts, irritability, and mood swings. There are a number of associated physical symptoms too, such as bloating, fluid retention, cravings, sore breasts, skin breakouts, insomnia, or difficulty sleeping. The idea that PMS is a condition requiring treatment is one I've questioned in recent years. In most cases, all that is required is allowing yourself the space to slow down and flow with your cycle. Embrace the opportunity for rest and make adjustments in your life as required to accommodate what your body needs. Some women do experience more intense PMS symptoms and even premenstrual dysphoric disorder (PMDD), an extension of PMS where usual life activities are severely impacted during the luteal phase. Usually symptoms improve when the period starts or within a few days.

Researchers still don't know exactly what is happening in the body during the PMS window to cause symptoms, but there are some leading theories involving progesterone, estrogen, cortisol, and inflammation. An insufficient rise in progesterone during the luteal phase may play a role in PMS, as progesterone has a calming, mood-elevating effect in the body. It does this by converting to a substance called allopregnanolone in the brain, which binds to and activates GABA receptors. Activated GABA receptors then release more GABA molecules. GABA is an inhibitory neurotransmitter, which means that it switches off brain activity, calming your anxious, stressed-out mind. Progesterone also promotes fluid balance, reduces inflammation, regulates the immune system, builds bones, and protects the heart.

Symptoms of low progesterone will occur when estrogen is too high, as the two play off one another in a ratio. Having high levels of estrogen is very common for women and may be a cause of heavy or painful periods. Note that estrogen is not all bad, as it helps to regulate some of our calming brain chemicals such as serotonin and oxytocin. The surge of estrogen prior to ovulation is one reason you experience a higher libido and increased energy levels and mood at that time.

Most commonly, failing to produce enough progesterone is a consequence of stress. Cortisol is produced from the same substance that makes progesterone. When we demand our body to divert most of this resource to cortisol due to the level of stress we are under, progesterone levels will suffer. Cortisol, a key part of the body's stress response, is more important from a survival perspective than the balance of reproductive hormones. The intensity of your PMS symptoms can act as a monthly scorecard, letting you know how well you have been managing stress. When your cycle is irregular, painful, or symptomatic in some way, it indicates that you likely have other systems in your body that are out of balance too. Most of the time, this is your body waving the white flag from ongoing stress.

We place such high expectations on ourselves, expecting our cyclical bodies to function like robots. We expect consistent energy levels, emotions, productivity, and motivation every day. As women, our cycles are very sensitive to stress, including physiological stress such as traveling overseas, physical injury, and interruptions to sleep. We're designed to devote significant amounts of time to rest, feeling our emotions, being creative, connecting to our senses, and slowing down. Many of us don't believe we have the time or lifestyle to accommodate this. Our bodies unfortunately will not adjust to modern life's expectations. Of course, it is impossible to avoid stress altogether and quitting your stressful job may not be an option. This is why supporting our bodies and keeping our hormones in balance with nutrition and herbal medicine is so important for managing PMS and the associated anxiety.

Supporting Your Hormones

You do not need to move to an ashram and become a monk dedicated to the path of enlightenment to have healthy hormones and reduce the hormonal roller-coaster ride of anxiety each cycle. Following are some key tips for keeping your hormones balanced even with the ups and downs of your stressful life:

- **Cruciferous vegetables:** Broccoli, brussels sprouts, cauliflower, and kale contain sulfur compounds that help the liver clear excess estrogen. Aim for two handfuls of these foods daily to support your hormones.
- **High-fiber foods:** Adding more fiber into your diet helps to clear excess estrogen that may be contributing to PMS symptoms. You should already have increased your fiber intake to support your gut microbiome, so this is an easy one.
- **Iodine:** This mineral may help clear excess estrogen from the body and supports progesterone. The best sources are eggs, seafood, and seaweeds like nori.
- **Magnesium:** This is another essential mineral that improves progesterone levels, balances estrogen, and helps the body to manage cortisol. You could add in a supplement, or consume

more almonds, black beans, cacao, dark leafy greens, and pumpkin seeds.

- **Track your cycles:** To start improving your hormone health, you must start tracking your cycles (if you are not already). There are many wonderful apps that can assist you with this. This will help you connect with your own patterns and figure out which phase you are in week to week. You can then adjust your schedule and expectations of yourself accordingly.
- **Vitex agnus-castus:** This is a herbal medicine that can reduce PMS symptoms by supporting progesterone production. Consult your healthcare practitioner to ensure it is right for you.
- **Zinc:** This is an important mineral for making more progesterone and managing PMS symptoms. You can take it as a supplement or eat more high-zinc foods such as almonds, chicken, chickpeas, hemp seeds, lamb, lentils, natural yogurt, oysters, and pumpkin seeds.

Practice

Use these guiding questions to start supporting yourself through your hormonal fluctuations.

- Do you need to track your cycles?
- Could you work on aligning your lifestyle with your cycles?
- Do you need to support your progesterone levels to reduce PMS intensity?
- Do you need to allow and invite in the ebb and flow of your cycle?

Perimenopause and Postmenopause

Anxiety around perimenopause is especially common, and it can occur postmenopause too. As menstrual cycles come to a halt, so does ovulation and the natural production of calming progesterone. Following the previous recommendations for increasing progesterone levels may be useful—namely increasing magnesium, iodine, and zinc. Body-identical progesterone therapy is another safe option to explore; this requires a prescription from your doctor. Compelling evidence is also emerging with research into the benefits of hypnotherapy for reducing anxiety in women postmenopause.[1]

Special Considerations for Men

Men's biology is much less complex when it comes to hormone fluctuations and anxiety. For most men under thirty-five, it is unlikely that levels of hormones such as testosterone influence anxiety. Low levels of testosterone may be a factor to consider if anxiety increases with age. Reducing alcohol intake, weight training to build muscle, and ensuring adequate protein intake and quality sleep are important for maintaining healthy testosterone levels.

Week Seven Checklist

This week there are two primary practices to play with. Let this week be full of joy and whatever feels good for you.

☐ Practice the art of pleasure by weaving pleasurable moments through your day.

☐ Apply what you have learned about your hormones, as required, to support yourself through any fluctuations.

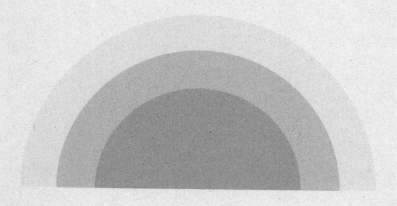

Week Eight: A Bright Future

The Scarcity Mindset

Have you ever noticed how much you live in a mindset of scarcity? The anxious mind will always tempt you into believing you don't have enough. It's another clever survival mechanism: If you err on the side of never enough, you'll be motivated to gather more resources that will keep you alive. Of course, most of us are not facing threats to our physical survival proportionate to the amount of time we spend worrying about not having enough. It has become the norm to talk about never having enough time. It's a trend to lament how busy we are. Social media is littered with memes joking about this theme. We're never doing enough or being productive enough. There's not enough sleep, friends, love, success, new ideas, or opportunities, and there's certainly never enough money. The more anxious you feel, the more scarcity thoughts tend to run rampant in your mind.

Spiritual teacher Wayne Dyer once said, "Abundance is not something we acquire, it's something we attune to." In other words, the literal number in your bank account can make you feel full of abundance or scarcity, depending on your mindset around it.

Practice

Where in your life do you feel there is not enough? Where does your anxious mind like to focus on scarcity the most? The aim of this activity is to bring awareness to your typical scarcity thought patterns, so that you can catch them and dismiss their validity more easily when they come up. Can you begin to notice how often you and others say there isn't enough?

Learning to Receive

To begin breaking down the well-worn scarcity thought paths, let's first take a look at how you feel about receiving. Many of the people I work with complain about not having enough money or support in their lives, but at the same time hold up their palm when help is offered. In other words, they resist the very thing they feel they lack. Do you feel guilty when asking for more in your life? Do you feel like you don't deserve more? Do you believe others will miss out if you receive more?

Consider the logic of this for a moment. We can all agree that the world is full of inequality and it would be great if things were fairer. However, does your guilt about what you have bring more to anyone else? Does feeling bad about having clean drinking water bring clean drinking water to those who don't have it? Guilt serves absolutely no one. It is simply a form of self-punishment: a maneuver of the inner critic that cuts you off from enjoying what you have. Isn't it the biggest slap in the face to those who have less than you if you ignore the opportunities and privilege you have? For you to sit there wallowing in your guilt and not do anything useful with your resources? Does guilt really motivate you to take action? Do you think you're the most effective version of yourself when you're operating from scarcity and anxiety?

What will motivate you to take the kind of action that will truly impact the world at the highest level is a feeling of abundance. Feeling confident and secure in what you have will have you asking better questions about what you can do to help the world from your zone of genius, using your unique talents and gifts. It will keep you from feeling overwhelmed by the burden of solving all the world's problems and shouldering all the challenges on your own, which will not get you very far. Trust me, I've been there—curled up in the fetal position on my bedroom floor, feeling absolutely helpless and hopeless because there is so much wrong with the world and I can't do enough about it. It took me a while to get over my own ego and to stop making my role in the world so pivotal. I had to feel abundant in my own resources, capable and secure enough in myself, to try anyway. Contributing a drop of goodness in an ocean of problems is enough. An abundant mindset—with an openness to receiving and pure appreciation, not guilt, for what you have—will allow you to live out a higher purpose on this planet. From this state, you have energy to give.

When you have met all your needs and your cup is full, you have more to give to the others around you. When you feel depleted and anxious, how does that impact the way you show up? When you're exhausted, how much patience do you have? When you are well rested, you can give so much.

When you were a child, did you notice that your caregivers resisted receiving too? How much did you as a child long for them to be happy and well rested? How much did you just want to see them in a state in which they could let go, laugh, and play with you? Perhaps you are a parent now, in a similar position with your children, or you may serve and take care of people in some other way. Remember, they just want to see you receive, fill your cup, and be happy too.

Finally, consider the joy you feel when you serve and give to others. It is a gift to allow others to experience the joy of giving to you too. Receive with a thank-you and a smile. Offer your heartfelt gratitude. Allow the other person to see that they have touched your heart. Surrender to the cycle of giving and receiving in life, just like breathing air in and out. Life wants you to breathe in as much as you breathe out. Allow yourself to connect back with this very natural way of being.

It is okay if receiving feels uncomfortable for now. It is currently unfamiliar to you. Let's make it familiar. It's really important that feeling comfortable with receiving is a priority for you—that you notice when you say no to an offering of support, a compliment, money, or some kind of assistance, and choose differently. Choose to allow it in. Say yes. Say thank you. This is the only way you can move out of your own way in reinforcing your scarcity beliefs and be the most effective, powerful version of yourself.

Mental Notes

- Your guilt or inability to receive from others does not bring more abundance to anyone else.
- It is a joy to give. Allow others the joy of giving to you.

Practice

Your new mantra around receiving is: "The more I receive, the more everyone benefits." Write this on your bathroom mirror or keep it somewhere you'll see it regularly. Repeat the words in your mind over and over this week. Whisper them when you wake up in the morning. Sing them in the shower. Write them in your journal. Let them steep in your soul like tea leaves until they become a part of you. Say these words as you carve out the time for yourself that you need so that you can continue to help and serve others around you.

Abundant Thinking

When you feel stuck and limited, like your life is so bleak and small that it could fit into a wooden box, I want you to practice abundant thinking. When anxiety shows up for me, it feels like thick clouds closing in around me, shrouding my vision. I can't see a way out. I can't see solutions. I start to doubt that there's anything more for me in this life other than what feels difficult, boring, or painful.

Back in my early twenties, in those years following the trip to Bali when my dad left my mom, I was deep in scarcity on every level. I already believed the lie that I was getting too old and time was running out. I know that sounds ridiculous, but the anxious mind is not rational. I was terrified that I'd never figure out money and achieve financial stability. I doubted my own capability to generate a secure income. I didn't believe in the infinite opportunities surrounding me. I literally thought I had to be a lawyer and that was the only way I could build a career that I would feel proud of and that would keep me afloat. I saw only one road to take. And yet, the idea of becoming a lawyer made me feel sick to my stomach. The one road I could take was not even really an option to me, because every fiber of my being rejected the concrete confinement and dull rigidity upon which the legal machine is built. A world where, from what I perceived, you are not allowed to be a human being. You have to wear heavy armor all day to hide your emotions, ignore your deepest needs (such as adequate sleep and regular meals), and become close to robotic to fulfill the demands of the work. My heart was calling me to an existence where I was free to express all my humanness, but I had no solutions. I didn't know how to do that back then. I was in anxious despair, stuck between two ideas: "There is simply not enough for me in this world" and "I am not enough for the world." Of course, this was all an illusion of my anxious mind—the illusion of scarcity.

There is a process to shift out of scarce, limited thinking and into a state of abundance. Here is how to do it. To step out of your scarcity box, start by being aware that you are in it. Say out loud to yourself, "I am in the illusion of scarcity right now." You'll notice that you are in scarcity thinking when all of a sudden it feels like there is not enough. The words "not enough" will come up repeatedly in the thought sentences of the mind, each time jolting you with another little dose of cortisol and adrenaline. You can affirm to yourself that these fears aren't as real as they feel. You can remember that the anxious mind loves to spiral into the irrational space as it tries to grasp for control. Just bringing awareness to this will help you to create some distance from the illusion, like you're stepping out of a thick fog you didn't even know you were in, and you can now figure out how to move through it.

Once you've identified the scarcity thinking, you can practice taking little steps toward expanding your mind into the beautiful, free-flowing state of abundance. You may need to unload some emotional weight before you can do this wholeheartedly. When the anxious thought cycle keeps repeating and the "stuck" feeling won't shift, you know your emotions need to be felt. I encourage you to bring in your loving parent to comfort your frightened inner child. This might look like having a cry or screaming into a pillow, or expressing your fears on paper to metabolize the anxious energy.

You're now ready to do the thought work of practicing abundant thinking. Go easy on yourself and choose a subject that's different to the one that feels most scarce. For example, if time and money feel limited, what feels abundant and easy to access for you? Perhaps thinking about the food available in your local area, all the different dining options, shelves of fresh produce in the supermarket, and coffee shops nearby feels easy. The ocean is a great abundant visual to anchor on to when you want your mind to expand out of its box. Focus on the immense volume of this beautiful body of water covering the surface of the planet. Take a moment to imagine the total number of cells in your body, each one of them operating miraculously, molecule by molecule, to keep you blinking your eyes, moving your limbs, thinking, talking, and laughing. Can you consider the sheer number of human beings alive right now, each one an entirely different character, living out their own unique stories and experiences? Each person with a tale to tell and something of value to offer this world? What about the limitless capacity for love in your heart and the hearts of every human being around you? You know that feeling when you thought you loved a person or a pet to the maximum, and then you reach a whole new level and it feels like your heart just exploded? New parents often say this about newborn babies. That's because there is no limit on love. Love is an energy that you generate within yourself, inspired by people, animals, experiences, and events around you. It grows with unlimited power.

Go broad now, working on the general feeling of there not being enough possibility, space, and openness in your life. You can use these abundant images and concepts to shift your focus to the limitless possibilities in your life, as countless as the cells in your body, yet to be discovered by you. What kinds of possibilities may await you, as far-reaching as the ocean, that you cannot even imagine? Think of the twists and turns your life could take and the unexpected wonderful surprises in store for you. You do not know what wonders await you. You do not know how your story will go. You do not know what you do not know.

Now return to considering the specific topic that feels scarce to you. You can apply this concept to money, time, dating, relationships, friends, or career opportunities, as well as the doubt you may feel around the likelihood of your deepest desires, hopes, and dreams coming true.

There is always more money to be made. There are avenues of wealth generation that you have not considered. There are valuable gifts within you that people would pay for that you have not thought about. There are other ways to earn a living besides a career in the corporate world. There are easier ways to make money than those you have discovered so far. Remember that money is a form of energy being exchanged, ebbing and flowing, constantly in flux. Less money this month does not mean less money forever. There is always more money to be generated.

Time is stretchy. Have you ever noticed that time flies when you're having fun, but a ten-minute meditation, sitting still watching your breath, can feel like an hour? Time is ultimately a concept you make up in your mind. It all comes down to how you perceive it and how present you are in the moment. Somehow no one has enough time, and yet we're all spending hours glued to our phones each day or bingeing our favorite shows on Netflix. There is time. You can always choose to make time for what is important to you.

When it comes to dating, it's easy to say from a scarcity mindset that there is no one out there. In this state of mind, you will swipe past thousands of faces, convinced no one will work for you. You don't need to find a catalog of eligible life partners lining up on your doorstep to feel abundant about the dating world. Remember that you only need one in a sea of hundreds of millions of potential partners. There are so many people who could be a great partner for you. Similarly, there are always new friends to meet—people with whom you share values and interests, people who would benefit from your support, care, and company as much as you would theirs. There are connections with people you have yet to meet that will enrich your life (at minimum) or completely transform it (at best).

In work, business, and career, there is always another path you could take. There is always a way of working that you haven't considered. There's always someone who could change everything by opening up your mind with one conversation. You have no idea what could be possible if you keep trying something and failing, and trying again. You can apply your skill set in ways you have not yet tried. You can always learn new skills and try new things.

Whenever you're facing a problem in life, when it feels like you're surrounded by brick walls and no options, remember this: You can't see the solution right now, but that doesn't mean it doesn't exist. You don't need to know exactly how things will work out to believe that it is possible. You don't need to know every step of the plan. You don't need to have it all figured out. You will find a way. The greatest message of abundant thinking is knowing that in this infinitely complex, amazing world, there is always a way. There is always more. You are free to breathe in the abundance. You were born to receive.

Mental Notes

- When you are in a state of anxiety, you are operating within a scarcity mindset.
- To shift out of scarcity, start by generally perceiving some ideas, thoughts, and topics that feel open, expansive, and abundant to you.
- From this more open perspective, you can start to see the scarcity topic you are stuck on through new eyes.

Practice

Challenge your scarcity thought patterns around the topics that feel most scarce for you using the process described. Write out a counterargument to each one. Take the time you need to contemplate your answer and put together the logical thinking that makes sense to you, so that your new abundant mindset can sink in.

Nourishing Your Future

Naomi moved back home to Melbourne after living overseas for five years. Nearing her midthirties, she was starting to feel desperate for a partner so she could settle down and have a family. She also had an amazing business idea that could take her out of her high-pressure graphic design work, giving her a mission and sense of purpose outside her personal life.

A few months after moving home, Naomi's confidence plummeted to a new low. She had been fired from her new job and told she wasn't reliable enough. A new man she had been dating for six weeks, the first person she had felt excited about in months, had stopped returning her messages. She was feeling on the outside of her friendships, with her closest girlfriends now consumed by motherhood and caring for their young families. The future looked like a big, empty hole; when she thought of it she imagined out-of-control doom and gloom. Her mind fed her a merry-go-round of thoughts such as "It's only going to get worse," "I don't think there are any good men left," "I'm going to die alone," "I won't ever become a mother," and "My best days are behind me."

I knew the feeling as she broke down in tears, describing the immense anxiety she was experiencing. Naomi was falling victim to a trick of the anxious mind that, left unchecked, has the potential to create crippling anxiety. Fortunately, together we could change this. We simply needed to create a bright future for her—one so real and vibrant that the worst-case disaster future couldn't carry such weight.

It requires conscious effort to nourish your future with images, ideas, and dreams that feel exciting, warm, inviting, and satisfying to you. You must do this consciously, because your mind will always default to feeding a future of doom and gloom where you expect the worst. This is a survival mechanism, helping you seek out potential threats with keen awareness so that hopefully you can plan, prepare, and prevent them from happening. If you automatically assume that something bad is going to happen, you'll be ready for the worst and more likely to survive. This works well when you're camping in the wilderness and you bring extra clothing to prevent hypothermia in case the weather forecast changes, or you take an umbrella when you go out, just in case it rains. It isn't so great when you're trying to control the big-picture future journey of a life that is pretty much completely out of your control.

At some point you have to come to terms with the truth: The only control you truly have is being aware of your mind, knowing the games it plays, and choosing what really serves you. You can live your entire life in fear, dreading the worst, suffering, and being prepared for disasters—most of which will never come to pass. Or you can live your life choosing to steer the content of your thoughts toward what will serve you, living each day in hope and positive anticipation for a brilliant life ahead. Even if the latter turns out to be false and the wonderful things you wish for never happen, wouldn't you rather spend your days in the feeling of hope than in anxiety, believing it's all downhill from here? It is the present moment and how you feel within it that matters most. The future is always at a distance. This moment now is the only moment you will ever exist in.

Picture your own unique doom-and-gloom future concept as a beast—a monster with gnashing teeth and bone-crushing jaws. In reality, this might be the idea of losing all your money, being left by your partner, something happening to your loved ones, getting a terminal illness, never having a family, or some version of being a failure. It is always hard to pinpoint exactly what you dread so much about the future. Try this now. Try to picture exactly what it is you're running from or trying to prevent from happening. Putting words to the feeling is a challenge, because there is little rational thinking, logic, or reason behind it. Now imagine that each time you consider another worst-case scenario or tell yourself you're going to die alone, you are feeding the anxious-future beast. You are nourishing the doom-and-gloom future vision, giving it sustenance and strength to perpetuate and penetrate your psyche more deeply.

It may soothe your mind to know that two researchers looked into measuring the percentage of worries that actually come true for people with anxiety. For thirty days, they followed a group of people with anxiety who noted down everything they worried about over a period of ten days. The study found that 91.4 percent of worries did not come true in reality.[1] This is further evidence that most of the anxious thoughts and worries of the mind are psychological junk not to be taken too seriously. Your worries are not as real as they feel.

Your work is to choose not to feed this anxious-future beast with more worries that aren't true and will probably never happen. You are essentially feeding yourself a series of lies. As the famous philosopher Seneca once said, "We suffer more in imagination than reality." How much are you torturing yourself with dark visions that will never come to pass? How are you taunting yourself with nightmare fantasies of your imagination that do not exist in reality? To take back your power and master your anxious mind, you must deliberately tell yourself better lies. You must make clear predictions about your future that actually feel good to you in this moment now, feeding your mind a future image that is bright, open, and hopeful. Turn your focus to starving the anxious-future beast by giving it less food and less attention. Instead, direct that energy and nutrition to a future vision that feels good.

Start building your image of a future full of light and beauty that makes you feel excited about where your life is going. What do you want to happen? How do you want to feel? Who do you want to be? Who would you like to be there with you? What thoughts, emotions, and feelings would you like to experience every day? If you get stuck on any of these questions, try asking yourself what you *don't* want, then identify the opposite of that and you'll have your answer. This is how you rewire your anxious mind: building a whole new vision of your life that excites and inspires you every day.

Practice

Write out a full page in your journal every day this week detailing your vision of your bright future as if it is already here. This is called future pacing. You'll write from the present tense as though you are living in that future moment right now. If you're facing a challenging situation, what would the future version of you say about how you overcame that challenge? Consider your work, family, friends, partner, health, hobbies, self-development, and lifestyle in general.

Here's an example:

I have just woken up and poured myself a cup of herbal tea, which I am sipping in my silk robe while listening to the birds outside in the garden. I feel peaceful as I muse over my contentment with where I am in my life. I look back on where I was when I started reading this book, and I can't believe the progress I have made. I am so proud of myself for implementing the changes I have. I've noticed lately that everything feels easier. Life is only getting better from here.

Making GABA

Did you know that there is a nutritional recipe for creating more of the calming chemical gamma-aminobutyric acid, more affectionately known as GABA, in your brain? This is as specific as nutrition can get when it comes to calming anxiety.

As you may have gathered from previous chapters, GABA has a calming, relaxing effect on the brain and the nervous system, slowing down brain activity as a key tool for the parasympathetic nervous system. GABA is your best friend if you want to help your body and mind relax. We all want more of it. You may have experienced the tranquilizing effect of an anti-anxiety benzodiazepine medication such as Valium, which works by facilitating the soothing activity of GABA in the brain. It's easy to form a dependence on benzodiazepines, though, and over time you need a higher dose for the same calming effect. It is not a suitable long-term solution.

Some herbal medicines help regulate the production of GABA in the brain and ease anxiety symptoms with minimal side effects or dependency risk. These are kava, valerian, hops, chamomile, Ginkgo biloba, passionflower, ashwagandha, skullcap, and lemon balm.[2] Some of these herbal medicines are not appropriate to be used with particular medications, in certain medical conditions, or during pregnancy and breastfeeding, so always consult your healthcare practitioner before trying them out. They can be used to break the anxiety cycle until you are in a place where you can cope and make the necessary changes you require to strengthen your Resilience Shield.

Your brain naturally produces more GABA when you trigger the vagus nerve and activate the parasympathetic nervous system. For example, when you lie down with your legs up the wall, the brain is releasing GABA. However, each time you do this, your body has to use up resources to make GABA. There are specific nutrient building blocks required to manufacture GABA. When the body has plenty of resources available, the production and release of GABA is far more efficient—and all the work you've done so far can be even more effective.

The nutrients that the body requires to make GABA are zinc, magnesium, vitamin B6, and protein. (I've included some information about how they work and an example of an effective daily dose on the following pages.) The amino acid chelate or bisglycinate form is preferred for minerals such as zinc and magnesium, as absorption into your bloodstream is enhanced. You can find this information on the supplement label, or ask your healthcare practitioner for advice.

Zinc

Zinc is an important mineral for many processes in the body, particularly in allowing for the release of GABA in the brain. You can take zinc as a supplement or eat more high-zinc foods such as oysters, almonds, pumpkin seeds, hemp seeds, chickpeas, lentils, natural yogurt, chicken, and lamb.

You may have a zinc deficiency if you have fingernails that break easily or grow slowly, you often get sick with a cold, or your sense of smell and taste isn't very strong. Plant-based or vegan diets are commonly low in zinc.

Example dose: 50 milligrams per day, with a break after two months to avoid impacting overall mineral balance. Always consume zinc supplements with food to prevent nausea.

Magnesium

This mineral can help increase levels of GABA by facilitating its production. You could add in a supplement or consume more dark leafy greens, pumpkin seeds, cacao, almonds, and black beans.

You may have a magnesium deficiency if you get aching muscles, you clench your jaw, your eyelids twitch, you experience period pain each month, or you can see a quiver to your tongue when you stick it out and look in the mirror.

Example dose: 500 milligrams per day.

Vitamin B6

This vitamin is also called pyridoxine and it works by acting as a catalyst for the enzymes that produce GABA. The best sources include pork, chicken, turkey, eggs, oats, brown rice, soy beans, most vegetables, and bread. Many zinc supplements also contain a good dose of vitamin B6.

Example dose: 20 to 40 milligrams per day.

Protein

Protein is made up of amino acids. Glutamine is a key amino acid that is used to make GABA while taurine is another amino acid that activates GABA receptors, allowing GABA to work better. You can find these amino acids in most sources of protein such as meat, fish, eggs, chickpeas, lentils, beans, natural yogurt, nuts, and seeds. Include a palm-size portion of protein per meal. Refer back to the Building a Calm Plate section in Week Six for more ideas of protein sources.

Practice

Consume a handful of sunflower and pumpkin seeds every day, as these are a great source of all the GABA nutrients. Alternatively, consult your healthcare practitioner to see which supplement may be right for you.

Week Eight Checklist

I've assigned you five practices in Week Eight. You may need to revisit the chapter to understand each practice in detail.

- ☐ Bring awareness to your scarcity beliefs and thoughts around where in your life there is not enough.
- ☐ Work with your new mantra around receiving: "The more I receive, the more everyone benefits."
- ☐ Challenge your scarcity thought patterns around the topics that feel most scarce for you.
- ☐ Write out a full page each day using the future pacing technique, detailing the vision of your bright future as if it is already here.
- ☐ Consume a handful of sunflower and pumpkin seeds daily to support your GABA levels.

Week Nine: Nurture with Nature

Dose Up on "Vitamin N"

Imagine you wake up in a white room. The sounds of the gray city rumble outside, but you hardly notice because you are so used to the concrete jungle in which you live. You spend hours of your day staring at a white screen, responding to emails and making calls in a white room, surrounded by white walls. It's after dark when you've finally finished work for the day. You contemplate whether it's worth going out for a walk. But it's cold outside and you're exhausted, so you turn on the heating and stay in—switching on the TV to unwind with a show.

It is all too easy to live life devoid of nature, or "Vitamin N" as I like to call it. That's why connection to nature is a key component of the Resilience Shield. The scene I've described may or may not depict the way you live your life, but it is no doubt a common story. Even if your situation is not to that extreme, there is likely limited time available in your busy schedule for sitting in a forest every day.

We are a part of nature, yet we have found so many ways to cut ourselves off from it. We need nature, yet we can go for days without seeing a tree, or, if we do, it's for a second before we glance back down at our phone. We are designed to live among nature, intertwined in ways I will soon describe. We intuitively know it is good for us. You will have experienced the soothing effect of a gently rippling river, the stunning blue of a far-reaching ocean, the impressive expanse of a mountain range, or the mystery of a whispering pine forest. These things draw us out of our mind and into the moment. Without seeing any science, we just know it is right to be in nature. Human beings have spent 99.99 percent of the seven million years we have existed in nature. I encourage you to make spending time in nature a priority in your life.

One thing I love about nature is the way it can teach us about life. As Albert Einstein said, "Look deep into nature, and then you will understand everything better." Nature is both the nurturing mother, soothing our nervous system with its rejuvenating qualities, and the keeper of life's wisdom. If you take a moment to sit in natural surroundings for long enough, with the intention of deep contemplation, you will uncover the secrets of life they have to share.

Nature teaches us that balance is natural. Everything in life seeks to return to a state of balance, whether it is the homeostasis in your body, the equilibrium effect of a chemical reaction, or the balance of your emotional state. When you give too much, you feel drained and cannot continue on in that way. If you don't balance out your giving with some receiving, eventually you'll burn out and be forced to stop and rest. Life will naturally bring you back into balance. If you don't choose your rest, life will choose rest for you. Too much work and not enough fun will leave you feeling flat, uninspired, and unmotivated. You are not made to be a productivity workhorse. Your most natural state is one of working and resting in a flow that feels good to you. If you overwater your plants, the roots will rot. If you don't water them enough, they will dry out. You cannot breathe out without also taking a breath in. The balance you seek in your life may appear to be out of reach, but if you tune in to the anxiety and address its message, you will find that shifting in and out of balance, being in a state of flux, is the most natural thing in the world. This is how nature breathes. This is life.

Everything in nature changes. With its revolving and evolving rhythms and cycles, nature helps us accept this fundamental beautiful rule of life. Through the year, the seasons move through summer, autumn, winter, and spring. Similarly, you are not designed to live in your summer state, striving for your goals at the top of your game, all year-round. Just look to nature for the permission slip you need to flow into your different seasons. In the constant evolution and change that takes place, you can also rest assured that no matter what you are experiencing, whether you are happy or sad, whether life is good or bad, it will all come to pass.

Nature teaches us that all is achieved in perfect timing. Picture the seedling rising up from the soil, slowly sprouting to life, growing millimeter by millimeter every day. Eventually, it matures into a thick oak tree. There are no deadlines or to-do lists in nature. There is no hurry to achieve or get things done, and yet somehow it all gets done. Everything in nature that needs to be accomplished is accomplished. Can you apply this concept to your life and the made-up deadlines you feel you must stick to and fret about? What about the timeline of your life—the idea that you should have done this by that age? What a beautiful way to live life instead, taking your time doing what feels natural to you, at your own pace, and allowing the rest to sort itself out—as it will. Nature teaches us to trust in the grand unfolding of our lives, in whatever form it takes.

Nature is the master of adaptation, regardless of the surroundings. Like the weeds growing up through cracks in the concrete, or the vine twisting around the railing, nature finds a way to adapt and thrive in any circumstance. How much time do you spend contemplating how to change your external world in some way—whether it's dreaming of a new house, a holiday, a fancier job, a better relationship, or a more fashionable wardrobe? Nature doesn't try to change the environment to suit it; it changes itself to suit its environment. It uses its inner resources to make the most of any external situation. The same is true in your life. You can always choose how you show up in your life. You can decide to adapt to any situation or challenge that comes your way.

Nature is powerful. Its profound strength and resilience is also in you. Plants and humans are made from the same stardust—the same atoms forming molecules that make up our cells. When we eat plants, they become a part of us. When we die, we merge with the earth that plants grow from. After a bushfire comes through, there is somehow still life in the charred trees. You'll soon see hopeful sprouts of green, striking and vibrant in the blackness. Nature's resilience is inspiring and it shines its examples all over the place. You just need to look for them.

Mental Notes

- Nature teaches that balance is natural, and change is the only constant.
- Nature shows how to adapt to the environment we are in, instead of trying to change it.
- Look to nature to remember that all is achieved in perfect timing.
- Nature reminds you of the resilience and power that are natural to you too.

Practice

This week, find a place in nature where you can spend at least an hour in quiet contemplation. It can be any kind of natural environment you like: a park, a beach, a forest, a desert, a riverbank, a cliff top, a grassy field, or a mountain. Allow your intuition to guide you to this place—somewhere you feel called to spend some time. When you're there, actively engage your senses. Take it all in with your eyes. Feel the textures. Breathe in the air. Don't rush as you arrive in your space. Walk slowly. Enjoy the stillness. You could bring your journal and write down your own lessons from nature as you sit there and immerse yourself in its nurturing, restorative energy.

Normal Is Unnatural

One of the questions my clients ask the most is: "Am I normal? Is this normal? Is that a normal thought to have? Is this a normal thing to say? Is what I'm experiencing normal?" What they are really asking is: "Am I doing it right? Will others approve of me? Am I fitting in?" Questioning whether you fit in the zone of normal is really about your sense of belonging and self-worth: If you belong, if you are normal, then you are a worthy human being. You get the tick of approval that you are doing life right, that who you are is correct.

If this resonates with you, I hope it comes as a great relief to know that there is no right way to live your life. Even the people who you really believe have it all figured out, absolutely do not. There is no set path or plan to follow. And you can't get it wrong either.

The concept of normal is completely unnatural. It's a made-up idea, created by human beings' anxious minds. The word "normal" only entered the English language around the seventeenth century, from the Latin *normalis*. This word was used by carpenters to refer to a right angle in a square. So, deep down, when we question whether we're normal, this is what we all want to be? A right angle? Sounds like a rather uninspiring pursuit to me. Look around at nature. Nature is not made up of only right angles, neat lines, and fixed categories. Nature is a vibrant jumble of different colors, textures, and forms. And it is stunningly beautiful. No one can argue that.

Yet we exist within a culture of set standards, expectations, and concepts around what is normal. Early on in life we learn what is considered normal and what is not. The young mind naturally seeks validation from guiding outside sources such as parents, caregivers, teachers, therapists, and other authority figures. Those who raised you wanted you to fit in and learn how to be a functioning member of society, so they taught you the rules of normal. Don't swear. Be polite. Groom yourself. Smile. Don't cry. Look nice for others. Control yourself. Don't talk about sex. Don't be rude. Be a nice person. Sit up straight. Be funny. Don't be weird. Make Mom happy. Make Dad proud. Get good grades in school. Just be good. Just be *normal*.

These rules are something we all adopt, whether they are stated explicitly to us or implied through action and values. The rules of normal start affecting us from before we are born. Nervously, two parents sit in the doctor's office, waiting for the all-clear that their baby is normal. Then we have normal ranges for growth and development, normal behavior and social skills to tick off, normal academic results, normal learning styles, and so on. For much of our lives we are positioned against the signposts of normal. Yet we live inside our flawed human selves, with "abnormal" swirly minds that think erratic, strange thoughts and feel uncontrollable, hurricane-like emotions. No wonder so many people think there is something wrong with them. None of us can measure up against normal. The idea that there is something wrong with you is one of the lies of the anxious mind, and now you can understand why and where you got it from.

You are perfection. You are nature expressed in human form. Consider that there are trees with smooth bark, trees with rough bark, tall trees, skinny trees, thick-trunk trees, and bent-over willowy trees. They all appear to be so different, and yet all trees are beautiful. You are just the same. Nature is full of unique beauty, and you are an expression of nature too. Your work is to let go of the misguided message that you need to conform to a standard of preexisting expectations. To do so is to deny the mighty force and power of nature running through your veins. Next time you find yourself asking "Is this normal?," remind yourself that this is a typical doubt of the anxious mind.

Mental Notes

- There is no normal or correct way to live your life, despite the pressure you may feel.
- To be completely normal and fit within a set standard goes against the rules of nature.
- Embrace the perfection and abnormal beauty of nature within you.

Practice

Can you normalize your experiences for yourself? When you are going through a challenging emotional experience like a wave of self-doubt or fear, tell yourself: "This is normal. I am normal. This is natural. I am nature. This is a natural expression." Can you normalize everything you say, think, feel, and do? If you can, you'll find you begin to accept yourself just the way you are, just as nature intended you to be. In that acceptance you will find a whole lot more peace.

Understanding Nature's Benefits

There are measurable, scientifically researched benefits to surrounding yourself with nature. We do not require clinical studies to believe that spending time in nature is good for us. We feel it innately. Yet it is fascinating to understand the myriad of ways nature positively affects our bodies. As you turn your attention to spending time in nature this week, consider just how powerful it can be for your overall well-being to be held by Pachamama (the Incan Earth Mother goddess).

Responding to the urgent need for more cost-effective mental health treatments, a group of researchers from the United Kingdom wanted to understand the impact of nature walks on depression and anxiety symptoms. They gathered data from cancer survivors, college students, and laypeople across the world experiencing mental health challenges, and found that symptoms of anxiety were consistently reduced from walking in nature.[1]

In another study, people who went for a ninety-minute walk experienced a drop in rumination—that unhelpful anxious thinking—and activation of the prefrontal cortex of the brain, which is involved in rational thinking and decision-making.[2]

Shinrin-yoku (forest bathing) is an established healing practice in Japan, in which people bring awareness to their senses while being immersed in nature. This is precisely the basis of your practice for this week. There is even a Japanese Society of Forest Medicine that conducts research on the therapeutic effects of forests on human health and provides education around forest bathing. Head researcher Qing Li says, "Wherever there are trees, we are healthier and happier." Research has shown increases in natural killer cells of the immune system that can help fight off infections and improvements in heart rate and blood pressure from forest bathing.[3] There have been numerous studies showing that forest bathing reduces anxiety, lowers cortisol levels, and activates the parasympathetic nervous system.[4] Spending twenty minutes in a park in the middle of a city is all that is required to have a significant impact on lowering your cortisol levels.[5]

So how does nature do this? Plants produce chemicals called phytoncides that have a calming effect on the nervous system as we inhale them. These chemicals are the antimicrobial essential oils emitted from the wood of trees and other greenery. There is also a higher oxygen content in the air in highly wooded areas that is thought to improve our mental state. Some researchers propose that being in an unthreatening natural environment is part of the de-stressing effect while others suggest that the sense of connection with nature can act as a proxy for our need for connection in general.[6] Another theory is that nature provides such an engrossing, rich subject for our eyes that it captures our focus away from rumination. Even looking at pictures of nature can produce a calming effect.[7] It is so essential that you bring mindfulness into your nature experience to milk the benefits. Looking at the greenery and inhaling the aromas mindfully is key for promoting a relaxation response. Consider all these ways that nature is nurturing you as you enjoy your nature time this week.

Vitamin D

Vitamin D is an incredibly important nutrient for a healthy, resilient human. Every cell in our body contains vitamin D receptors, suggesting that it plays a role with each cell in some way. We need to be outside in nature, exposed to sunlight (taking the required precautions of course), to create vitamin D. Imagine how well plants would grow without sunlight? Human beings are nature too.

Vitamin D is actually a hormone, not a vitamin. It helps to regulate your immune system, may reduce your risk of diseases such as osteoporosis, encourages DNA repair, supports your hormone balance, and plays an important role in robust mental health. Adequate levels of vitamin D in the body are associated with less anxiety, less depression, and better sleep quality. It helps the brain to regulate levels of calming brain chemicals like serotonin and dopamine.

If your skin does not see the sun daily (even in the cooler months), or you wear a lot of clothing or work indoors, it's likely you are not getting enough sunlight to make the optimal amount of vitamin D.

Those with fairer skin tend to need less time in the sun to produce the optimum amount of vitamin D while those with darker skin require longer periods of sun exposure.

Vitamin D supplements are also available and are helpful if you can't spend much time in the sunlight. The form of the supplement is not so important here.

Example dose: 1,000 to 4,000 international units per day.

Practice

In addition to your time in nature this week, also spend a few minutes per day with your arms, legs, and chest exposed to the sun unprotected to support your vitamin D levels. Be mindful not to burn your skin, and adjust this recommendation to a shorter time frame according to your needs and skin type. Consider taking a vitamin D supplement if required.

Iron and Oxygen

Iron deficiency is incredibly common in menstruating women, as they are losing blood from their bodies every month. Iron is required to make hemoglobin, the magnet center of a red blood cell to which oxygen attaches. Without adequate iron levels, oxygen can't be carried easily to your cells. Oxygen is energy for cells (including brain cells) and without it, they can't function. If brain cells are not functioning, that can cause anxiety, brain fog, difficulty focusing, decreased motivation, poor memory, and low energy levels.

You also need iron to efficiently make serotonin, as it is involved in the chemical manufacturing process. Iron is a regulator of GABA in the brain, helping to balance out an overstimulated, anxious brain.[8]

For women in particular, there is a significant correlation between iron deficiency and risk of anxiety and depression.[9] While correlation does not equal causation, given the important role this mineral plays in the day-to-day functioning of your cells, it is well worth considering in your arsenal of anxiety resilience. While there is no specific research to show that supplementing iron to correct a deficiency will reduce anxiety, there is research that suggests correcting an iron deficiency can reduce the risk of mental health disorders more generally.[10]

Iron is found primarily in red meat, such as beef, lamb, or pork. I recommend grass-fed for higher omega-3 content. Tuna, chicken, dried figs, apricots, almonds, cashews, hazelnuts, pine nuts, sesame seeds, tahini, eggs, parsley, cacao powder, dark leafy greens, coriander, spinach, spirulina, and silverbeet are also good sources. Note that animal-based sources are more bioavailable for the body, meaning the iron is more easily absorbed than with plant-based sources. It is important to consume a mix of animal and plant-based sources, unless you follow a specific diet in which this is not possible. If you are vegan, vegetarian, or rarely eat red meat, a daily supplement may be your best option. You'll need regular blood tests with your doctor to monitor your iron status. If you are a menstruating woman and you have no idea where your iron levels are sitting, I recommend you have a blood test to check.

The ideal supplement form for iron is the bisglycinate form, which is gentler on the digestive tract and more easily absorbed into the blood.

Example dose: 24 milligrams per day.

Practice

If you haven't had your iron levels checked within the last twelve months, it's time to visit your doctor for a blood test. Ideally your ferritin (the storage form of iron) levels should be above 50 nanograms per milliliter. If you are below this level, you may need to take a supplement and increase your intake of iron-rich foods.

Week Nine Checklist

In Week Nine, I invite you to connect deeply with nature with four practices.

- [ ] Find a place in nature where you can spend at least an hour in quiet contemplation. Actively engage your senses.
- [ ] Practice normalizing your experiences this week. Can you start to accept yourself just as you are?
- [ ] Support your vitamin D levels with sun exposure (taking appropriate precautions) and supplements if needed.
- [ ] Have your iron levels checked and, if needed, consider taking a supplement and increasing your intake of iron-rich foods.

Week Ten: The External World

Creating a Calm Environment

Most of this book focuses on finding control where it really exists: within you. This is the one section where we'll examine the external environment and how it can influence the way you feel. At the end of the day, your external circumstances are neutral and you can always choose the story that you tell yourself about them. You can feel better in any environment using the power of your thoughts. Equally, if you can change your circumstances to improve your life according to your preferences, of course you should.

Have you ever noticed the way your house becomes less organized and more of a mess the more anxious you feel? As you start feeling better, naturally you start to put the clothes away, clean the dishes in the sink, and vacuum the floors. And you might also notice you feel better while you tidy things away, as though the physical tidying process is helping you organize your emotions and thoughts. A tidy home supports a tidy mind.

The famous home organizer Marie Kondo says, "The space in which we live should be for the person we are becoming now, not for the person we were in the past." So take a look around you. Consider your bedroom, your kitchen, your living room, and your bathroom.

Look especially closely at the places where you store things—the old stuff you hang on to, *just in case*. What is your space saying about you? Who is this space for? What adjustments could you make to create a space that nourishes your nervous system and brings a smile to your face?

Are you surrounded by bright colors that feel warm and uplifting, or are the colors bleak and dark? Could your space be more organized? Are you allowing your space to be filled up with stuff you don't need—stuff that feels heavy and unnecessary that you're holding on to unconsciously? Is your house a warm, spacious sanctuary, or a storage space? Take a look at your digital stuff too. You will be surprised at what you keep stored in photos, videos, and old conversations in the cloud that no longer need to be held on to.

If you have trouble letting go of these things, ask yourself, "Why is that?" Get curious with yourself. What does it mean for you to hang on to it, and what does it mean to let it go? Is this stuff truly benefiting you, or does the frightened little child within you feel safer surrounded by stuff? Are your things a safety blanket, reinforcing that inner child's habits and behaviors, keeping you stuck in old patterns? What does that little child need to hear to feel safe with or without the stuff? Do you, as the adult you are now, need these things in your life?

As you explore these questions and move around your space, coming across different objects, you'll notice before you reflections of many of your old behaviors and choices. The impulse purchase you made to cheer yourself up and push down the sad, empty feeling. The photograph you can't throw away, because you wish the person in it was still here. The old journals, scrawled, tearstained pages like relics of your pain, that seem so important and needed—but you actually never go back to read through them now. Each object symbolizes something. Each one is a message to your subconscious mind about who you are.

In my space I like to keep an indoor plant, rough-cut crystals, or giant shells from the ocean, as I love nature. I make pleasure a priority through the scents I collect in candles, oils, and lotions. I have beautiful tools around me that remind me to slow down, like my Tibetan singing bowl, cozy blankets, and books full of wisdom. I use warm colors like gold, peach, and pink that brighten the coldest of days. The things in my space make me feel good. They reinforce my values and reflect back to me who I am becoming.

What does your space say about you? Who are you becoming? What could you surround yourself with to reflect this?

Mental Notes

- If you can change your environment to better your life and make it more enjoyable, I encourage you to do so.
- The things you surround yourself with in your home usually symbolize something about you and can influence your subconscious mind.

Practice

Use your home environment to make purposeful statements about who you are becoming. Does your space reflect your values and who you are becoming? What changes need to be made? What are you still holding on to in your space? What could you let go of? What could be tidied, cleaned out, mended, upgraded, or organized? Can you make space to invite in a new chapter of your life? How can you put more of *you* in your space? Write out your answers to these questions and make a list. Set some time aside this week to make it happen.

The People Around You

While the key message in this book is to work within your true sphere of control rather than wishing helplessly for others to be different and behave the way you would like them to, we cannot ignore the fact that life is full of people. People will provoke you. People will hurt you. People will poke at your wounds. There are many people you have and will encounter who will do things you don't like, say things that upset you, and behave in ways you wouldn't dream of. There are people who cannot be pleased, people who cannot be reasoned with, and people who manipulate. The people around you provide a perfect setting for triggering anxiety. You have to find a way to somehow live in this world peacefully among them. The pursuit of remaining content and empowered within yourself despite the people around you is one of life's greatest opportunities for growth. If people didn't challenge us, we wouldn't grow. With this being said, how on earth do you deal with the people around you?

Every person you contact can have an impact on you, particularly the five closest people in your life. Taking a look at these five people can even predict your future: There are things that may be predetermined based on statistical probability about what will happen to you in your life based on who you spend your time with. This information can be worrisome, I know, but it is equally empowering. When you know better, you can make informed choices that lead you where you want to go.

This idea that the people around you influence you is called social influence. Nicholas Christakis and James Fowler were the first to study social influence using data from the Framingham Heart Study—an ongoing study that began tracking 5,209 adults from Framingham, Massachusetts, in 1948. According to their results, if a close friend of yours becomes obese, you are 45 percent more likely than chance to gain weight over the next two to four years.[1] While I do not want to incorrectly imply that obesity is simply a matter of food intake and exercise when it is in fact more often rooted in trauma, this remains a powerful example of how social influence works. In my family growing up, no one was overly athletic or sporty. It's not that no one moved their body at all, it just wasn't a key identity—like some families who would go on hikes on the weekends, play in all the sports teams, or enter fun runs together. It seemed unusual to get sweaty on a daily basis. Restful weekend mornings in front of the television watching reruns of *Friends* were normal when I was a teenager. Even now, when I work out around family members, I feel the social influence as they comment that I might be overdoing it, or even how impressive it is. I'm always reminded of the norm that I am pushing against the zone established in my family group—and the belief that "We are not highly active people." Building the habit of regular exercise became like walking up a path with an incline for me. It was not as simple as remembering to take nutritional supplements like fish oil, for example. My mom started giving me fish oil capsules to swallow after breakfast when I was in elementary school. Taking supplements is a natural, easy, downhill slope for me. It's normal in my family group.

The influence of a social group is not by default negative, Christakis and Fowler reassure us. Surrounding yourself with happy people makes you happier too. If you have a friend of a friend of a friend who is happy with their life, you have a 6 percent greater likelihood of being happy yourself. Now, 6 percent may not seem like much, but put into context it is actually rather impressive. If you were to receive an extra $10,000 raise in your salary, this would only increase your happiness by about 2 percent. It also shows you just how powerful the ripple effect can be when you make a positive change in your life to create more contentment and satisfaction yourself. It will influence those around you. While the saying might be true that hurt people hurt people, healing people heal people. When you actively do the work yourself, you are making a positive impact on the people around you.

Your social community has an influence over you and the anxiety you experience. It's time to take an inventory of that community, bring some awareness to it, and make changes if need be. There is no need to cull your entire social circle overnight or cut ties with family members unless of course they are harming you. This is a process. As you become more aware and notice behaviors that don't feel good to you, you might slowly distance yourself from certain people, creating boundaries and spending less time with them. You might choose not to answer a phone call or make plans with that person. You do not have to be friends with people you don't like. You don't have to make time for people who drain you. Perhaps you will spend more time instead with people who do reflect the values you possess and the kind of person you are becoming.

Practice

Who are your five closest people? Write down their names. Take some time to contemplate their traits and habits. Are they supporting your growth or hindering it? Do they reflect your values and who you want to be? This is not about judging or criticizing others or placing blame. This is about becoming aware of the impact the people around you have on you.

How might other people be contacting you and entering your space, influencing you in ways that do not serve you? Consider the emails and messages you receive and the social media accounts you follow. What boundaries do you need to create? Do you need to unsubscribe, mute, block, or unfollow?

Next, consider who is the most confident, grounded, calm, and positive person you know. Do you know anyone who already possesses many of the qualities and values you are working on moving toward? How can you spend more time with this person? Where do these kinds of people hang out? Are they at yoga classes, wellness conferences, or health retreats? Are they already friends with your friends? Are they going to women's circles, meetups, or self-development workshops?

If you do not have direct contact with people like this in your life, allow people who inspire you to enter your life in other less direct ways. Listen to their podcasts, read their books, and follow them on social media. Immerse yourself in the energy of uplifting people who already embody who you wish to be, and deliberately absorb their positive influence. You will naturally start to become more like them. Over time, you will notice more and more people who embody these values appearing in your life.

Boundaries and Saying No

Do you ever find yourself feeling resentful, like everyone is taking you for granted and no one is really listening to you? Do you feel unappreciated and like people just walk all over you, taking advantage of your kindness and generosity? If so, this is a big sign that you need to work on your boundaries. Resentment, often coupled with anxiety, is a signal from your body that your boundaries are being crossed. Even if you've done this kind of work before, reviewing your boundaries is always relevant, as these personal rules are ever-evolving.

Boundaries are the rules you set that govern your world and how others behave within it. Your boundaries are determined by you and only you. They are informed by your past experiences, your moral compass, your customs and culture, your sense of the right way of doing things, how you wish to be treated, and how you treat others. They are different for everyone. No one can tell you that your boundary is silly or unimportant. It is up to you to decide. The interesting thing about boundaries is that we automatically assume other people have the same ones. We think, "Why would you treat someone like that? I would never do that." We get upset and fret that someone else has different boundaries. But of course people will have different boundaries and that is okay. That is their right. Your job is to assume they do not know your boundaries and you must kindly bring them to their awareness. When someone knowingly and intentionally crosses your boundary, that's another story.

Have you ever offended someone without realizing? You would hate to walk into someone's house with shoes on when it's a shoes-off kind of house. You need someone to tell you what is and isn't appropriate. Imagine standing in someone's living room, noticing their face harden as they look down at your shoes that you haven't removed. You have no idea what you're doing wrong, but you feel like you have upset them somehow. It's not your fault that no one told you what the rules are, and you would have appreciated being told. When you know the rules, you feel comfortable in another person's house. So, if you feel uncomfortable about speaking up about a boundary, remember that it's a kindness on your part to share that boundary with the other person.

If you don't set boundaries, people will walk all over you. They'll encroach upon you. You will end up a resentful people-pleaser, feeling disempowered. You will have less to give, less energy, and much more anxiety. When you say yes to everyone else, you are essentially saying no to yourself. You must learn to say no to as many people as it takes to avoid saying no to yourself. This is part of living a more authentic, aligned life where you are the master of your anxious mind.

You are not a bad person for setting a boundary. The most compassionate people are actually those with really strong boundaries. These people have the space in their hearts to feel more compassion for others, to step out of judgment, gossip, and petty arguments, because they protect their energy. They simply have more to give. They don't let everyone encroach on their energy. You probably know the feeling of being too exhausted to remember to bring in your inner loving parent when you need it. When you have strong boundaries, you can readily practice compassion for yourself, allowing you to be a great person to be around.

Keep in mind that setting boundaries is not about getting other people to change how they behave around you. What other people do is not a marker of your success in setting a boundary. People get to do what they want and you have no control over that. You do get to choose how much time you spend with people who do and don't respect your boundaries. The important part is that you've made a clear declaration about your self-worth. Ultimately, it's about improving relationships, feeling respected, and becoming closer to those who do respect your boundaries.

You know you need to set a boundary when someone does something that creates a tense, belly-sinking feeling within you. You will know it when you feel it. Just imagine right now how you would feel watching someone walk into your clean house wearing muddy boots and put their feet up on your new white linen couch. That's the feeling. It might feel like anxiety, or like frustration, anger, disgust, or resentment. That's how you know a boundary has been crossed and it is time to speak up. It's time to say, "That is not okay with me."

There is an art to expressing boundaries. Bear in mind that you do not need to have the perfect dialogue here, but using these guidelines can help you feel more confident and supported as you become more familiar with this practice. The main goal is that you attempt to communicate your needs in a situation where you would normally hold back and let a boundary be crossed. Say it even if you feel mean. Say it even if it feels unnaturally direct. Say it even if it brings up anxiety for you.

State the Intention

It can be helpful to begin by stating the overall intention of what you have to say, which may be that you want to support, nurture, or improve this relationship in some way. You could say, for example, "I'm bringing this up because I want our relationship to be the best it can be."

Offer Appreciation

Depending on the person you're speaking with, you might next offer some words of appreciation for what they do that pleases you—something you admire or respect about them. This instantly takes the defensiveness out of the interaction. For example, "I probably don't say this enough, but your commitment to your career is really admirable."

Make a Request

Next, you can state your boundary in the form of a request. The art of boundaries is all about crystal-clear communication. You need to provide clear instructions around how you would like this person to behave in future, even if it seems obvious to you. You could say, "I really need your help to keep my house clean. Could you take your shoes off first before walking inside?" Another example could be, "I'd love your help in finding a solution, but I can't continue this conversation when you speak to me in that tone," or "It would work a lot better if you could put down your phone and look at me when I need to share something important with you." Another way to make a request could be letting someone know how their actions make you feel and the consequences of this by saying, "When you do this, I do this." For example, "When you walk in with muddy boots, I feel like you don't respect me and I shut down. Can we change that?" It is not enough to just tell them that what they do upsets you. Do not stop with how you feel. Feelings are murky and confusing for other people without a clear request.

Alternatively, Just Say No

Don't forget that stating a boundary can also be really simple. It can take one sentence, or even just one word: no. You might say "That doesn't work for me" or "It would work better if…" or "This makes me feel uncomfortable." You're communicating that something doesn't feel right for you about this interaction and removing the potential for resentment. It all depends on the situation and you'll sense when a longer conversation is required.

Please prepare yourself that the closest people in your life, like old friends, partners, and family members, will often be unsupportive of your new boundaries. Expect this. They're used to you passively saying yes to all their demands. These are the people who benefited from crossing your boundaries in the past, thinking, "Oh, she'll be fine with it." So when you start standing up for yourself, some conflict may happen. Expect to feel uncomfortable. It's all part of the process and evidence that you are growing. Each time you see them react, be proud of yourself. Congratulate yourself for defending your self-worth.

Some people might try to make you feel bad about it and call you selfish. I have had that same objection from my family too. What's important is that you know you made the right decision for you, and you bring that inner loving parent in to remind you that you are a good person. You know you are coming from a place of wanting to have energy, capacity for compassion, better relationships, and something to give. You are doing this because you don't want to simmer away with resentment, which ultimately damages your most precious relationships.

Your family member, partner, or friend only rejects you putting yourself first because they don't uphold their own boundaries. It's kind of like "Well, this isn't fair, I don't get respect for myself." It is not your obligation to stay at this same unconscious level, as much as I'm sure you might love them and want them to grow. None of this makes your family member a bad person. They are just human, and they're not coming from a place of empowerment themselves. Maybe they never will, but you still can.

Mental Notes

- A boundary is a rule you set that governs your world and how others behave within it.
- If you do not set boundaries in your life, people will take advantage of you and drain your energy.
- A successful boundary being set has nothing to do with how the other person responds. The important part is that you had the self-worth to set it.

Practice

A boundary is a rule you make for how you want to be treated. Write a list of your boundaries. What behavior will you accept and what won't you accept in your relationships? What is okay and what is not okay? What are you available for? What aren't you available for any longer?

The Genetic Influence on Anxiety

Have you ever wondered how genetics influences anxiety? Much of it comes back to methylation, which is controlled by your genes. Methylation is a series of essential chemical reactions that occur in every cell in the body. Your cells are methylating right now as you read this. In these chemical reactions, a methyl group is added to DNA, proteins, and other molecules, like the brain chemicals that improve mood and calm anxiety.[2]

Methylation can positively or negatively impact a number of different processes in the body, including your heart health, hormones, liver detoxification, DNA repair, immune cell production, and inflammation. Problems with methylation have therefore been linked to recurrent miscarriage, dementia, heart disease, cancer, mood disorders, and autoimmune diseases.[3] Your susceptibility to methylation problems comes back to your individual genetic variants, some of which may impact anxiety. If you have any of these issues in your medical history or they run in your family, further investigation and addressing problems with methylation becomes much more important as it is more likely that your genes are involved.

It is estimated that 20 to 40 percent of people carry a genetic polymorphism on the gene MTHFR that can slow down the process of methylation in the cells.[4] There are many different genetic variants that can impact methylation, though, so do not place too much weight on MTHFR if you do have it. Keep in mind that everyone has different combinations of genetic variations, just like we all have different strengths and weaknesses. If you do not have a genetic polymorphism that impacts methylation, or any link to the previously listed conditions, you likely do not need to take this part into much consideration.

If you feel there is something wrong, you can test for methylation issues by visiting your doctor, naturopath, or another healthcare professional to check your levels of homocysteine. High homocysteine usually suggests that methylation is not working very well. I recommend that you have your active B12 and folate levels checked too, the reasons for which you'll soon understand. DNA testing is available to see if you have any of the genetic polymorphisms that can make you more prone to issues with methylation. Note, though, that your genes do not bind you to a specific health outcome in the future. Genes are simply markers that tell you what issues you might be more susceptible to if you do not take care of yourself. Genes are the computer program, but you are hitting the keyboard to turn those genes on or off with the way you eat and live your life. You have a lot of power over your genetic destiny.

Keeping methylation running smoothly is simple: Manage your stress, exercise regularly, and eat a whole-food diet with plenty of B vitamins. Do these things and methylation should not be too much of a concern for you. If you eat a mostly unprocessed diet with an abundance of greens, quality meats, eggs, lentils, nuts, and seeds, you are getting a broad spectrum of the B vitamins you need. Vitamin B6, folate, B12, and B2 are particularly significant. Consult a healthcare practitioner to discuss whether supplementation is right for you.

Vitamin B12

A deficiency in vitamin B12 is linked to anxiety. B12 deficiency is much more likely in those who eat a vegan diet, as this vitamin is only found in animal-based foods or produced by bacteria. Algae such as spirulina is one of the rare exceptions that contains vitamin B12, but unless you want to add spoonfuls of a substance that tastes like pond water to your meals, a supplement is a good choice.

Sources include: cheese, chicken, eggs, fish, grass-fed red meat (beef and lamb), milk, pork, tuna, and yogurt.

Folate

You will likely get enough folate most of the time if you eat whole foods in your diet. Folate is essential for a healthy pregnancy, and it is also linked to improving symptoms of anxiety and depression when a deficiency is corrected.[5] This is one reason why people feel better quickly when they start eating more whole foods.

Sources include: all vegetables, dark leafy greens, grains, and meats.

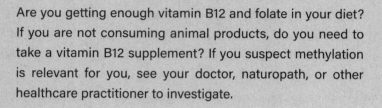

Practice

Are you getting enough vitamin B12 and folate in your diet? If you are not consuming animal products, do you need to take a vitamin B12 supplement? If you suspect methylation is relevant for you, see your doctor, naturopath, or other healthcare practitioner to investigate.

Week Ten Checklist

You have four key practices to explore in Week Ten. Refer to the relevant sections of this chapter for guided information.

- ☐ Tidy, clean out, upgrade, and organize your home environment to reflect who you are becoming.
- ☐ Complete the practice assessing your five closest people. Then consider how you can bring more positive, grounded people into your life.
- ☐ Write a list of your boundaries.
- ☐ Consider the role that genetics and methylation may play for you and support yourself nutritionally if required.

Week Eleven: Healthy Emotional Expression

Sleep for Balanced Emotions

How do you feel when you wake up in the morning? Are you waking through the night? Do you find it difficult to get to sleep, with your mind often ruminating? Is sleep a priority in your life? Quality sleep is part of the Resilience Shield and is essential for building anxiety resilience. Your brain is primed for anxiety when you do not get enough sleep, or enough high-quality sleep. This is something that still affects me now. When I've had a poor sleep, I know that the anxiety I feel is a physiological response in my body. My brain knows that my body is in a compromised state without adequate sleep, so it switches into high-alert mode for protection. The technical term for this is anticipatory brain function. Knowing this takes the blame away from you and shifts the experience of anxiety to one that is expected—and easy to correct with a better sleep the next night.

One night of sleep deprivation impacts brain function equivalent to a blood alcohol reading of 0.05 to 0.10. The brain is so hungry for the nourishing dream state of rapid eye movement (REM) sleep that when we don't sleep, we start dreaming while awake. We can hallucinate. Lack of sleep impairs memory and information processing. It causes the brain to increase anticipatory reactions—a survival mechanism that has us anticipating potential threats to our safety. This keeps us looping in doom-and-gloom future thinking and anxiety. The brain chemicals that keep us feeling calm and maintain a stable mood are also disrupted. So how can we optimize our sleep for stronger anxiety resilience?

A Regular Bedtime

Try to maintain regular sleep and wake times every day, varying by no more than an hour or two. Your body's cells thrive with a regular schedule each day. How often might you be disrupting your cells' circadian rhythm by sleeping in for three hours longer on a Sunday morning? We accrue a kind of jet lag called social jet lag from staying up late and sleeping in on the weekends. That's not to say you can never shift your sleeping patterns, but keeping this in mind and trying to keep them relatively even can make a big difference.

Sleep Away from Your Phone

Create boundaries with your phone. Turn your phone to airplane mode while you sleep to minimize notifications coming through in the night and your temptation to pick it up. A phone screen is very stimulating to the brain. It's designed to capture your attention in every way with its bright colors and the promise of another dopamine hit keeping you coming back for more. Reducing your screen time in the evenings is a good idea, particularly from 9 p.m. onward, as this will help you produce more melatonin (the sleep hormone). Screens produce a blue light that can interrupt your body's melatonin production and stop you from feeling sleepy. Phone use will also wake you up when you are trying to sleep. The jury is still out when it comes to the impact of electromagnetic frequencies emitted from phones on sleep quality, but there is plenty of evidence to suggest that keeping your phone close by while you sleep does reduce your sleep quality and increase the likelihood of experiencing anxiety.[1]

Keep Cool, Dark, and Quiet

Keep your bedroom low in temperature and completely dark. Your eyeballs are able to detect light even when the eyelids are closed, sending a signal to the brain that the sun is still up or starting to rise, even in the middle of the night. Keep pets and children out of the bedroom as best as you can. Use an eye mask and earplugs to improve your sleep, blocking out excess sounds and light.

Create a Wind-Down Routine

You may like to create a wind-down routine if you've noticed your sleep quality has declined. This means setting a half-hour window of time before bed after you've conducted all your chores and hygiene tasks like brushing your teeth. Your routine may include dimming the lights, journaling, lying with your legs up the wall, reading a book, inhaling lavender essential oil, meditating, or stretching gently. Taking a bath or a hot shower before bed can help you get a great sleep: your body temperature rises and then cools, naturally sending you into a sleepy state.

Other Factors to Consider

Here are some more factors to consider when it comes to sleep:

- Alcohol and caffeine affect your sleep quality and should already be something you are only consuming in moderation, with awareness of their effect on you and your anxiety resilience.
- Avoid eating dinner too late; if possible, don't eat within two hours of bedtime.
- Get some sun and expose yourself to bright light during the day so that it is very clear to your brain when it is daytime and when it is night. Your brain needs to have that connection to the sun to regulate its sleep hormone cycle.
- If you struggle with sleep, avoid stressful activities like work and exercise well before bedtime. Do not exercise within three hours of bedtime.
- Limit your intake of liquids within an hour of going to bed, so you are not waking up for the toilet through the night.

Nutrition for Sleep

Some foods may improve sleep quality by supporting your melatonin levels, allowing for a deeper, more restorative sleep:

- **Almonds and walnuts:** Snacking on almonds and walnuts may help you sleep, as they are natural sources of melatonin.
- **Kiwifruit:** Another study showed that adults with sleep issues who consumed two kiwifruit before bed had improved sleep quality.[2]
- **Oily fish:** In one study, those who ate 300 grams of Atlantic salmon three times per week for six months fell asleep on average ten minutes faster than those who ate only chicken, beef, or pork.[3]

- **Tart cherry juice:** There is research demonstrating the sleep benefits of consuming tart cherry juice, another source of melatonin.[4]

Practice

Do you need to make sleep a priority? What changes could you implement this week? Experiment with the suggestions here and see if they improve your sleep quality and strengthen your Resilience Shield.

Anxiety at Specific Times of Day

Have you ever noticed that you experience more anxiety at different times of the day? For some people this happens almost like clockwork. You may experience more anxiety just after waking or in the evening before sleep. Both morning and night anxiety tend to stem from a feeling of dread about the day—whether it's a day about to begin or a new day that has to be faced on the other side of sleep. Here are some strategies to get started.

Morning Anxiety

Understanding that there is a natural rise in cortisol in the mornings has been a great help to many of my clients. Cortisol rises in the morning to wake you up and get you started on your day. It gives you a burst of energy and alertness that can easily be perceived as anxiety. If you've trained yourself to panic as soon as you notice the uncomfortable, restless sensation in your body, you'll then start a cycle of anxiety. You might think, "Oh no, I'm anxious! There's something wrong."

I recommend that you instead relax into the feeling of alertness upon waking, reminding yourself that this is just a rise in cortisol to wake you up. Your body is doing its natural thing to help you wake, and you're doing your part by allowing this process to happen. Tell yourself, "This is normal. I'm feeling a rush of cortisol and that's a great thing. It tells me my body is healthy and in balance. Isn't my body wonderful for helping me get started for the day?" As you do this, you soften your response to the anxious feeling. You can then bring in the tuning-in practice to soften the experience even more.

The next thing I recommend is resisting the urge to pick up your phone for the first fifteen to thirty minutes of your day. This gives your brain a chance to wake up slowly and orient you to the new day. You can spend this time taking a shower, meditating, dancing, engaging in physical exercise, or stretching your body. It's easier to detach from your phone if you leave it charging overnight out of reach and away from your bed, such as on the other side of the room or in a different room altogether.

Don't linger in bed. Get yourself up fairly soon after you've woken up, as the longer you linger, the more time you have to ruminate and worry about the anxious feeling.

If you do all this and you're still feeling anxious, you might find you need to express your deeper underlying emotions, speak to your inner child, or question the unconscious fear-based stories moving through your mind about what this day will bring. Journaling in the morning can be a good way to do this.

Night Anxiety

If you're experiencing more anxiety in the evening, you may find you're subconsciously afraid to sleep and face the next day when you have to do it all again. Or you may have a sense of not having done enough for the day, and therefore not feel you can allow it to conclude with sleep. In addition to the sleep recommendations previously discussed, there are some additional supports for anxiety at night.

The first thing to do if you're tossing and turning and unable to sleep is to get out of bed—especially if the cycle is growing with momentum. If you share your bed with a partner, get up and move to a different room. Turn on dim yellow-orange lighting to protect your melatonin production and engage in some relaxing activities like reading, stretching, or journaling. Lighting that looks like candle- or firelight is closer to what our ancestors used in the evenings, and it does not interfere with your levels of melatonin. Do not use a device or screen. Blue light from screens and any other white-blue lighting at night can reduce melatonin production and result in a poorer sleep. Moving to a new location and removing the pressure of needing to fall asleep right now helps to interrupt the thought cycles that fuel the next wave of anxiety. Once you feel sleepy, you can return to bed.

Implementing a wind-down routine and practices to trigger the vagus nerve to move into rest-and-digest mode can be helpful. A specific practice I recommend for bedtime anxiety is getting out your journal and writing down everything you're worried about. Start with the sentence, "I can't sleep and relax right now because…" and let the words flow out of you from there. This might lead to writing up a plan for the next few days and scheduling in time for each task, so that you can see how everything that hasn't been done today will be done. It might look like questioning your thinking. This is also a great time to bring in your inner loving parent. Remind yourself—just like the most incredible, compassionate parent would—that you've done enough for today, and you've earned a restful night's sleep. Reassure yourself that all your problems will work out somehow—you simply don't know the specifics of how that will happen yet. Right now, at this time of night, in this emotional state, it is not the optimal time to figure out the solutions. Trust that they'll come to you after a good sleep, when your brain is actually able to reconfigure information and come up with creative solutions. That's what a great night's sleep does. So solve your worrisome problems by inviting sleep to take place.

No matter what time of day you typically experience anxiety with a greater intensity, these solutions are mostly temporary supports. Working with your Resilience Shield and the guided practices in this book will provide the deeper change you are seeking.

Letting Go

For so long I held on to the story of blame and anger toward my dad. I was addicted to it. It soothed me in a way, to feel some power in such a powerless state, to feel so much certainty in my own rightness and his wrongness. I could not allow his betrayal to be okay in any way. He had to be punished for the hurt he had caused. However, I believed that life wanted me to expand beyond this event, using it as a catapult to more freedom and love, beyond my mind's fears. There were many more gifts of joy the Universe was sending my way.

A few years after that trip to Bali I found myself sitting on a beach with my journal and a book in my hands. The book was a self-development classic: *You Can Heal Your Life* by Louise Hay. I shuddered with bitterness as I became aware of a wedding taking place on the foreshore behind me. My dad was getting remarried in a few weeks. My heart was closed, fused only tighter shut by the happiness radiating out from the nearby ceremony. In my state, I couldn't be happy for others. Not if it triggered me, poking at my painful wound. I couldn't feel joy. I couldn't let in the love that was all around me. I was blind to the lighter side. The beauty of life only pushed me deeper into my pain. Staring out at the ocean, I turned to the chapter on letting go. With a long sigh, I realized I was blocking my own peace.

Letting go is not about saying what someone else did was acceptable in any way. Please note, there is no need to engage in this practice if it does not feel helpful or desirable for you in your personal healing journey. You're invited to consider where you can release past hurts a little more. This practice is about releasing yourself from the burden of holding on to a story that weighs you down and has you giving your power away to another person. There are people you have encountered through your life who you are holding on to, like I was. You might not think about them regularly but somewhere, in the depths of your mind, those grudges are there, gathering weight as psychological junk. If that person shows up in your life, or someone brings them up in a conversation, or you are reminded of them in some way, you'll find your mood changes. Your energy will drain away and you'll be left feeling unsettled. Anxiety has been triggered.

Holding grudges can keep you feeling small, like you don't deserve more in life. It reinforces the self-harming belief that life is against you—that you've been wronged, and that another person can come along and steal all your light and power from you. The truth is, you remain powerful no matter what you experience.

We all have many people who we need to release. We collect them as we go through life. The high-school bully who humiliated you, the guy who rejected you at the party, the ex-partner who cheated on you, the sister who criticized you, the friend you fell out with, the boss who didn't pay you enough, and so on. You get the idea. The list of grudges grows longer and pieces of your power become more scattered and dispersed into each one of them.

Considering your situation, is there someone obvious who comes to mind that you need to have a conversation with—even if only in your head? Is there someone you have unfinished business with, who you need to write a letter to that you'll never send? If there is, you may feel called to take the steps to release them this week as an act of love for yourself. There is by no means any requirement for you to complete this practice in order to move forward as we all have unique experiences, but many people find this useful. It is up to you to decide whether it will be valuable for you and you may like to work privately with a therapist to guide you.

As you consider those who you'd like to release, can you see that this person has had failures, pain, fear, and suffering in their life, too? Can you see that this person learned their behaviors, beliefs, and ways of being from somewhere else? This concoction of a human being and what they did is a tragedy of humanity as a whole—the bittersweet symphony of life itself. And so, can you feel pity for this person? Can you take off your mind's fogged-up glasses and connect with your true self?

Practice

Write a letter to yourself. In this letter, write the words, "I let go of..." followed by every person's name and each action they took that you can think of. When you can't think of anyone else, write, "I forgive myself..." and allow the words that need to flow. If emotion comes up for you during this process, allow those feelings to be there.

Emotional Body Work

If you want to feel better, you have to get better at feeling. It is very common for me to see clients who struggle to express their emotions. If this is you, you might feel like there is a wall up or a blockage when it comes to feeling. Even those who would say openly that they cry a lot, or cry easily, often aren't allowing the space to fully release the emotion. If you believe you are too sensitive, too emotional, or too much, you may find yourself trying to pull yourself together sooner than you are really ready to. You don't feel deserving of taking up the time and space you need to really sit with your feelings. There is a subtle holding-in of the tears all the same.

Emotion is energy in motion—a stormy gray cloud passing through your blue sky. Emotions naturally move through a process like a wave through the body, gathering momentum, peaking at the top, and falling away. However, most of the time we do not allow the emotional wave to come forth. We shove our feelings down and force ourselves to work, distract from them, and numb ourselves with food, alcohol, online shopping, social media, recreational drugs, or other addictions.

When sadness, fear, and anger are not expressed, these emotions are not released. When they are not released, where do the emotions go? Emotions that are not released remain inside your body, storing up with energy. That energy feels uncomfortable, restless, and contained in the body. It leaks out of you anyway, like a dam overflowing with water, the walls shuddering with the pressure. The restlessness of unexpressed emotion is what we often call anxiety.

In some cases, this energy builds to such an intensity that it erupts from us, more like a volcano, into a panic attack or depression. The good news is that this doesn't have to happen if you can become more comfortable with allowing yourself to feel.

If you want to explore where your resistance to feeling fully comes from, ask yourself: What happened when you expressed emotion when you were growing up? Did someone tell you that it was wrong in some way? Was the wrongness of emotional sensitivity implied without words by the people around you who never let you see their emotions? Was there anyone to demonstrate to you what healthy emotional expression looks like? When you were upset, were you told to just get over it, or smile and be happy? Who was there to help you when big feelings came up, teaching you how to ride the wave of emotion safely? Most of us were not given adequate support when it comes to expressing emotion.

To effectively release your emotions is to release stress and anxiety from your nervous system, bringing yourself to a natural state of calm. Through shedding tears or screaming out your feelings, you lower your body's cortisol levels, release opioid pain-relieving chemicals, and activate the parasympathetic nervous system. It's a process of allowing your feelings to be there, accepting your humanness, and letting yourself feel when you need to (and you will need to often). Grief is a lifelong process. It is not limited to a six-month period following the death of a loved one. There is always something to grieve as we move through constant change and loss. This does not mean you should dwell in the depths of sadness all day every day; in the moments when sadness does show up as the sting in your eyes, the heavy feeling in your chest, or the ball in your throat, see if you can make space for it to come forth and release.

There are other ways you can shift emotion without forcing yourself to cry and needing to shed tears.

Breathwork

Breathwork is a powerful way to let go of that heavy energy and access deep layers you have been suppressing. You may choose to explore a deeper journey through attending a breathwork class led by a trained facilitator—these are held monthly in my online programs—or you can try some breathing practices on your own. Right now, wherever you are, you can try a simple box breathing technique to calm your nervous system. You simply breathe in through your nose for the count of four, hold for the count of four, breathe out for the count of four, and hold again for the count of four. You can repeat this process for a few rounds for as long as you need. You could also try the reset breath, where you set a timer for one minute and breathe in and out through your mouth, lips in an oval shape, at a relatively fast pace—like you are power walking. Use enough force that you could blow out a candle. At the end of the minute, hold your breath for as long as you can. You can repeat this for three rounds. There are many other breathing techniques to explore, some of which can last ten to thirty minutes. All will leave you with a profound sense of calm.

The Pillow Scream

Screaming into a pillow is another potent emotional release exercise. It helps you access the anger that often sits on top of sadness. Find a private space where you can commit to this with your full capacity. You may find that after three or so screams you feel the urge to cry rise naturally. You can also punch the pillow and grip it tightly with your hands, allowing the wild fury inside you—the rage of generations of oppressed people before you—pour out. Focus on the injustice, the unfairness, the people who have wronged you and treated you with disrespect. This might be people you are close to, or distant figures in society who enrage you. See their faces and speak to them as you scream. I encourage you to scream louder than you think you need to and really put some energy into it, channeling the deep anger that society may not allow you to express. This practice works well for people of all genders, but I've found that women (and those who have had their voices oppressed) find it particularly healing. If a woman is shown to be angry, she is automatically labeled as crazy. Women don't want to look crazy, so we hold it in. This is your opportunity to claim back your power and do it anyway. Be loud, take up space, make noise, and let it out.

Mental Notes

- Emotions are a signal that energy needs to move. If you do not move it, it will leak out of you as anxiety or erupt in a panic attack.
- Releasing your emotions is releasing stress from your body. It's good for you!
- Every one of us needs to make space for grief in our lives. We must allow the sadness to flow as we say goodbye to people, places, animals, and parts of ourselves that we love over and over.

Practice

Lean in to your emotions and give yourself permission to feel them. If you let yourself have a big cry this week, allowing all the space you need to get to the bottom of the emotional wave, that is even better. Try the breathing and pillow-scream techniques described here.

Week Eleven Checklist

In Week Eleven, there are three important practices to implement. Refer back to the descriptions in the chapter for a more detailed explanation of each one.

- ☐ Experiment with optimizing your sleep and make sleep a priority in your life.
- ☐ Write a letting-go letter, listing the names of those you need to release, as well as the things you need to forgive yourself for.
- ☐ Lean in to your emotions and give yourself permission to feel them, using the techniques described.

Week Twelve: Choose Your World

Trusting in Life's Journey

What would it be like to fully trust in your journey through life? Take a moment to feel into this idea. When you trust in life, you give your full presence to enjoying what is in front of you in each moment. You are awake to your senses. You drink in all the juice of life around you. When something appears to go wrong or is different than your preferences and expectations, you are peaceful. You know that something better is always in store for you. You delight in the next opportunity for growth. When the path turns wildly around a shadowy corner you hold on to your hat, trusting that this road is always in your favor and comes with everything you need. You live in a state of blind faith every day, knowing you are being led to something greater than you can imagine.

A challenge arises. You trust. You land the job of your dreams, but after three weeks you're made redundant. You trust. You meet The One and plan your whole life together, but after three years, the relationship falls apart. You trust. The brand-new apartment you bought a month ago floods. You trust. You're finally pregnant, only to lose the baby at ten weeks. You trust. You get a scary health diagnosis and the odds are against you. You trust. Your favorite person in the whole world passes away too soon. You trust. You see war, financial crises, natural disasters, and pandemics on the news. You trust.

I have lived through many of these challenges myself. If I haven't lived them directly, I've met those who have and worked with them. Somehow, no matter the stretch of the imagination required, I promise that the peacefulness of trusting the journey is always available to you.

I met someone who I thought was the love of my life. Just over a year into our whirlwind international romance, I quit my job, sold my car, paid thousands of dollars for a visa, and moved to the other side of the world to be with him. I was convinced we would be spending our entire lives together. When our relationship didn't work out, I sank into one of my deepest challenges in the game of trust since I began this inner work. The grief pulled me down into days of zero appetite where I saw no point in leaving my bed. My heart was shattered. The ache was so physical, like a real wound I had to nurse. I wished I could have wrapped it in bandages or applied a numbing salve, but all I could do was cry it out until the ache in my heart was replaced with an ache in my head. All I could do was surrender to the process, and remind myself not to fight and struggle against it. For a while, every day my mind kicked and screamed against the wrongness of it. There was a part of me that very much felt I had been left out in the dark. Part of me felt forgotten about by the Universe, like maybe all my dreams for the kind of life I wanted were foolish. And yet, at the same time, I trusted.

Naturally, I dipped in and out of the trust as my future plans dissolved into gray confusion. My mind would spiral into fear for hours before I could catch it and land back in my heart again. But I did catch it. I was amazed that through my heartache, in the darkness, I could still hope with such intensity too. It was how I imagine it would feel to skydive out of a plane with a cocktail mix of terror and thrilling joy. I would whisper to myself, "I can't see it now, but this is working out for me. Somehow. I still get to live a wonderful life, with or without him in it. There is more that I can't see. There must be more. There must be something even better." I must have written words to that effect over a hundred times in my journal in the weeks and months that followed. I imagined myself telling this story one day—how it might help someone else. I made it my mission to prove my hopeful perspective true, to prove that I could trust in the hidden gifts that this devastation would eventually bring. I thought a lot about the way those green bursts of new life sprout from the blackened trees after fires burn through. I trusted in my rebirth. I trusted in the wisdom I would gain from the pain. I trusted in what I did not know, beyond the limits and lies of my anxious mind. I trusted in life surprising me yet again with a beautiful twist I didn't see coming, in equal measure with the painful turns it doled out. I trusted in the uncertainty stretching before me—not as the emptiness it was so easy to perceive it to be, but as a blank canvas waiting to be filled with color. And I trusted in the person who was holding the paintbrush. That was me.

Anxiety is at its core an inability to feel comfortable and safe in life. When it comes to working with fear, finding some way to trust in the wild roller-coaster ride of life is essential. You must craft a belief system that serves you in this endeavor. Martin Luther King Jr. once said, "Faith is taking the first step, even if you can't see the whole staircase." But how do you trust in an unpredictable world that has hurt you, thrown you one too many curveballs, and taken loved ones from you? There might be monsters at the end of that staircase. How do you take a step when the rest of the stairs are hidden? How do you relax on this ride of life when it may also traumatize you and leave you all alone in the dark?

There is no answer other than to surrender to and trust it. You trust that even if there are monsters, you'll have what you need to fight them or move away from them. You trust that pain and challenge is temporary and ever-evolving. You trust that growth is beneficial, and you do not grow when you are comfortable. You trust that, ultimately, everything that happens in life is neutral. Whether it's good or bad depends on the meaning you give it. It is all about the story you tell.

There is something about the mental game of figuring out the neutrality of our life events—balancing the tragedy with hope, no matter how devastating the situation, how deep the trauma, or how uncomfortable the pain—that lights a fire in me. I have used this to navigate my own life challenges countless times and I guide my clients to it too. I love to ask: "How can this too be working out? Where is the good in this bad? What am I not seeing right now? What is the glimmering star in this black night sky?" It may well be the most rewarding and uplifting part of my work. So far I have never failed to find a gift in any painful, tragic circumstance. There is always something of value gained. It may take several years for the value to show itself fully, but it is always there.

Your mind is an alchemist; instead of turning metal into gold, it can transform your pain into beauty. In my case, in the present moment as I write this book, a dream of mine for so long, I genuinely would not have wished for my story to go any other way. It has taken time, grief, inner work, and shifting perspective to get to this place of authentic trust. I have gained all that I held out hope for in those dark moments—and more. There was so much more for me—more than my limited mind could have imagined—waiting to be discovered. Life was always working out for me, as it is working out for you.

Mental Notes

- To trust in the journey of life is to go through disappointment after disappointment and keep asking the question: "How is this still working out for me?"

Practice

Can you assign yourself the mission of finding the gratitude, the spark, the light, and the hope in something that has felt bleak and tragic in your life? Can you really test the limits of your imagination and ask yourself: "How was even that situation working out somehow? What if that is possible even in a tragedy like this? Where was the value in that experience?" If you have the patience to work through this and be open to that possibility, eventually, I promise, you will always find it.

Overcoming Trust Issues

I was once convinced that none of this was true. I grew up in a family of atheistic lawyers; believing in anything more than what the mind can rationalize with solid scientific evidence was not exactly encouraged. After I left high school and started finding my feet in the big wide world, I found an empty space in my heart. I was longing for something to believe in, somewhere to rest from my fears and the cold, bleak reality of life's tragedies. As a child, I loved to play pretend and create worlds full of magic in my imagination. Transitioning into adulthood, I still felt that need to connect with magic and wished to place my faith beyond what the eye could see. I was jealous of the people who went to church on the weekends, not only for the community they had, but for their unwavering belief that after death there is heaven, and that someone is always looking out for you. It is my personal opinion that as humans, we need to believe in something greater than ourselves in order to be at our highest level of health, well-being, and mental resilience. I felt the lack of it in my life as a quiet yearning, the seeds of a deeper knowing that there was more than *this*. Perhaps you can relate to that feeling.

The older I get, the stronger my faith becomes. The more I experience life, the more I gather evidence of the rocky moments working out just fine. The more I allow negative emotion to wash over me, the more I trust in the glorious relief on the other side. I no longer fight the contrasting dark moments, so the light comes back to me more effortlessly. The more I delve into gratitude for what I have now, instead of clinging to what I may lose in the future, the more content I feel in life. I have deliberately crafted a belief system that serves me. And, I realized some time ago, this is not nonsense. It's not naive. It makes perfect logical sense to do so if you want to master your anxious mind.

Perhaps there are things you already believe in, a faith system you already subscribe to that you don't even realize counts as believing in what you have no evidence for. It could be believing in the law of karma, that what goes around comes around; that good and bad luck exist; that some things are just "meant to be"; the rules of astrology; the idea of fate, that things happen for a reason; the influence of the moon; mind-blowing psychic predictions; even soul mates. It could be more obvious, like practicing a religion. Or perhaps you have your own ideas around whether or not there is a god, and what God even means. You might believe in your spiritual self and your connection to Source, the place from which everything we have in this world comes. It could be that through your meditation practice, you've discovered entire worlds to explore within yourself. You already know you are more than your mind's thoughts. You are the observing presence watching the stream of thoughts. It requires a level of faith to tune out the outside noise and surrender inward. And so, chances are, you do believe in *something*. It is so human to feel compelled to follow this calling toward trusting life, even when there is no rational reason for it.

As you already know, the story we tell about our lives is what creates our reality. We are all living in a delusion of some kind, viewing the world through a narrow lens of past experiences, social conditioning, and beliefs. It's all a lie. It's all a story. You can choose to believe in the delusion that you are the victim of your life, alone and singled out to suffer. Or you can tell a story that serves you and empowers you, where the Universe has your back and always provides what you need to grow and develop through life along your chosen path. If you are going to live within a delusion, at least choose one that is helpful. The most convincing part of the argument for me is not about whether or not this belief is fundamentally true and evidence based. What inspires me to dive headfirst after trust in the Universe is knowing that if I tell this story about my life, I will *make it true*.

If you have a dream to work for yourself and build a business based on your creativity, and you believe that the passion stirring in your heart was gifted to you for a reason—that it's a sign of the Universe's desire for you to bring your creations to life—are you more or less likely to give up when it gets hard? If you tell yourself that the first ten people who tell you *no* are just bumps in the road, and you feel confident that the Universe will bring the *yes* to you when the timing is perfect, are you more or less likely to eventually hear that yes? If you don't really have the money right now for the next logical step, but you believe if you take a risk and invest in yourself, the Universe will always provide you with everything you need, are you more or less likely to win? No doubt, the talent in you must be there to meet these opportunities, but talent is nothing without opportunity. And where did your talent, your gifts, your intelligence, and your genius ideas come from in the first place?

When you believe the Universe's will is on your side, you take bolder actions, you show up with more confidence, you become magnetic to others, you see more possibilities, you ask for more, you create more opportunities, and you make your own luck. You do not stop when it doesn't go your way. You are resilient to failure. You keep going until you get to where you want to be. You trust that life is guiding you through a process to get what you want, or leading you to a destination even better than the one you had pictured.

You have a choice. You can disregard the superpower you have of trusting the Universe and telling the story that builds your confidence and lights your heart on fire. You can stick to the science-only approach. You can stay in the safe, controlled world of data and numbers. But science is just a language to translate magic. We know there are sound frequencies we cannot detect with our human ears. We know through quantum physics, looking inside atoms at the electron level, all the predictable Newtonian rules of how matter behaves go out the window. We know there are mysteries in this universe we will never be able to solve. Do you really think your fearful mind knows more than the infinite intelligence of the Universe that created you? Who are you to think you can predict the worst outcomes for yourself in a world that is so complex and ever-changing? Who are you to believe that this life is more heavily oriented toward bad outcomes, pain, and tragedy? Who are you to declare that you know better? Who are you to say you cannot trust in the journey of life?

Trusting that the Universe has your back is one of the wisest decisions you can make in your life. You are most welcome to keep on telling the limited, fear-based story that all there is in this life is what you can see. Buy in to the delusional fear of all the other minds that surround you. I won't stop you. I will, however, wake you up to the limitation of that approach. When it comes to what's possible for you in your life, to believe in what you have no evidence for is to make a very clever, intelligent decision for yourself. It is to activate a power within you that allows your full potential to come to fruition. You will find that your life becomes a whole lot more interesting and much more fun.

Explore what happens when you follow that tiny spark of hope in your heart. See what happens when you feed that hunger inside you for a belief in something to lie back into and hold you safe. Let all of life in, including the infinite intelligence of the Universe. If you wish to feel free, direct the focus of your anxious mind with the stories you tell yourself about this reality and take a leap into all that is possible.

Mental Notes

- To be at our highest level of resilience to the knocks and challenges of life, human beings require a belief system of some kind.
- You are telling a delusional story about your life, whether you've based it on what you can see and touch or not.
- If you're going to live in a delusion, you might as well tell a story about your life that serves you.

Practice

Could you experiment with this idea of taking a leap of faith for a week or a month, just to see what happens? You don't have to stick with it. You can go back to the old way if you want. Why not just play with this? Consider something you'd really like to create in your life, and trust that if you take action steps forward, one logical step after another, telling yourself that you're supported in this process, it will work out for you.

It might not work out exactly how you expect. It might not include the exact circumstances you think it needs to. But you can certainly create the essence of it. Everything you think you would feel by having this amazing creation come to life is possible, because the feeling of having it is the only reason you want it anyway.

For example, if you want a new car, what you really want is freedom and excitement—the luxurious feeling of sitting in the leather seats and the satisfaction of driving on a highway with the sunroof down and your favorite person next to you. It's not about the car. It's not about the money. It's not even about the specific person. It's all about the feelings you wish to feel. And you can have it all.

Choose Your World

You have the power to make your world as safe, wonderful, beautiful, and exciting as you want it to be. So let's play with this. Life can be such a game when we make it that way. Chances are, you've felt like the game has been playing *you* for too long. Wake up to the fact that you're the one making the rules. You've allowed this game to play you by believing in a delusion that doesn't serve you. What would happen if you decided to believe that the Universe is on your side? What would it be like if you trusted that life was supporting you and working out for you? It is time to select a perspective on life that serves you and start choosing your world. You are no longer a slave to the external circumstances around you. You are taking back your power.

The expectations you set for your future determine what happens next for you. Similar to our practice of future pacing in Week Eight, you are setting yourself up to fail or succeed based on what you tell yourself an experience will be like. When you decide that there is no option and no way it can work out well, that is what you will experience. You'll look for the evidence that proves your story true.

Let's say you're feeling nervous before a social event. You imagine everyone there will be more impressive and more beautiful than you. You are already anticipating their judgment of you as inferior to them. Anxiety is buzzing around in your chest. But hang on, you haven't even met these people yet or arrived at the event. This is all a made-up projection in your mind. If you think this way, as you arrive at the event you will automatically look for the judgment in people's eyes. You'll perceive them thinking, "She sounds like an idiot when she talks." You'll be biased to your own delusion, and you will feel even more uncomfortable. You'll have no idea if any of what you think is true, but you're *proving* it true: that you're someone who doesn't belong in this place.

Whatever you are experiencing in your life that isn't desirable to you, such as a boring job that makes you dread your week, *you* are contributing to the perpetuation of that undesirable situation by believing there's nothing you can do about it. You are living in a state of learned helplessness where you've felt so beaten down and disappointed in life that you no longer even try to change it. You give up your power without a second thought. You say, "Oh well, there's nothing I can do." And so, without meaning to, you are choosing this for yourself and allowing it to continue. That's the world you are choosing for yourself.

To change this, you must ask yourself what kind of world you'd like to live in. What kind of work life would you like to experience? Even if there's nothing you can do about your situation right at this moment, no doubt it feels better knowing you are now actively seeking change. Doesn't it feel good to step out of the helplessness into something more powerful? Practice opening your mind to the possibility that you can do this differently, that any undesirable circumstance can be altered in your favor. It all comes back to the meaning you make of the situation and where you focus your attention.

What would happen if you chose to focus on the elements of the job that you do find tolerable, or perhaps even enjoyable? Maybe there is a coworker who has become a really close friend and gives you a satisfying feeling of connection each day. Maybe the paycheck arriving in your bank account feels really good. Maybe there's something about signing off at the end of the day that helps you feel like you've accomplished something.

What would happen if you changed the story? You might be telling yourself something like this right now:

I'm stuck in this soul-sucking job forever. It's literally killing me. I can't stand the thought of doing this one more day, but I have to pay the bills. I'm just feeling so trapped in this. There are no other options. I can't leave, because the job market is terrible right now. What am I going to do?

Could you start telling the story like this, instead?

Right now, I am in the perfect place to ask for more of what I do want in my career. I've never been clearer on what I don't want to experience. I'm going to use the power of directing my focus to see what is working for me in this job. I'm going to find gratitude for the things that are going right for me. I'm also going to ask for more. I'm in the process of working this out, and I don't need to have it all figured out right now. One thing I'm sure of is that I am on my way to something better, because life is always working out for me. My eyes and ears are now wide open to all the possibilities finding their way to me, some of which I've never even imagined before. I am so excited to see where this new path leads me.

When you decide that there are always options you're yet to uncover and that things are always working out for you, that is what you will experience. You will take off the veil you've had over your eyes, blocking you from seeing clearly, and orient your focus to seeing the solutions. You will allow answers in. You will let yourself see what is already going well for you. Your excitement for this quest in your life for better, while being grateful for where you are, will have you bringing it up in conversations. You'll mention it to someone, maybe at a social event where you confidently tell the story that you're going to meet some really lovely humans that night who really click with you. You'll discover this person you're talking to is looking for someone just like you to take on a role in their company, a job that lets you travel the world and even pays more than your previous position.

It's a role that gives you all the freedom and excitement that you're craving, that your other job didn't offer.

Now, these written words can only teach you so much. You will have to experience this in your own life to drop into trust as you gather your own evidence and deepen your faith. But there is one thing I'm certain you'll discover: This is how the game of life works. You are so much more powerful than the anxious mind has had you believe. You can choose to live the life of your dreams. Now that you know all this, are you willing to play?

Practice

Choose a day this week to simply decide that people are going to be really kind, warm, and friendly toward you. Choose this experience for yourself. Write down a few sentences of what it might be like to go through your day with such warmth from people. Keep this intention at the forefront in your mind throughout the day. Look around for the smiles. Expect to see kindness from strangers. Expect to see people outstretching their hands, offering to help you. Expect to see evidence of good, loving humans. When you look for it and set the intention, you will experience it. This is a great starting point as you gather more evidence that it works and deepen your trust. Keep setting positive expectations and looking for what you want to see. Soon, you can ask yourself where else you'd like to see change. You can move on to choosing other elements of your world to shift in your favor too—be it your health, wealth, career, or love life.

Gratitude for Anxiety

You are almost ready to complete this healing journey with me. The final stage is feeling thankful for the painful, challenging experience of anxiety that you intended to transform when you started this work. Mastery of the mind is seeing all sides of your experience through life. It's knowing that anxiety is not merely a symptom to cure. It is both the wound and the source of healing. Anxiety has brought much wisdom and growth into your life. Can you feel into that gratitude for the anxiety and the role it has played in your life now?

Could it be that your anxious mind has been calling you toward a much more trusting relationship with the Universe? Could it be that anxiety has brought you closer to magic, closer to expanding into all the possibilities that await you in your life? Could it be that anxiety has led you to make changes that have given you better health? Could it be that anxiety has helped you be kinder and far more loving toward yourself, acting as a reminder when you falter from serving yourself at the highest level? Could it be that the anxiety has led you to grow into the best version of yourself, one that can overcome fear and see through the limits of the mind? Could it be that anxiety has brought you deeper into faith that the Universe does have your back, that you are guided, that you are safe, and that you are so loved?

Could it be that anxiety has been looking out for you, calling you back to your truest self all along?

Anxiety is a sign of being out of alignment with what is true for your highest self. It's a sign that you can trust, that you *should* trust. You do not need to separate from this safe knowing anymore. Anxiety is the navigation system of your life, telling you when you are moving away from where you really want to be. It is time to thank anxiety for everything it has brought into your life.

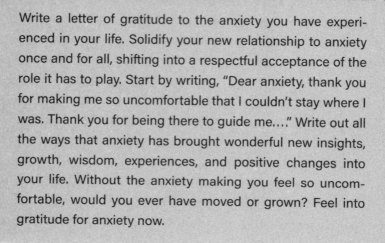

Practice

Write a letter of gratitude to the anxiety you have experienced in your life. Solidify your new relationship to anxiety once and for all, shifting into a respectful acceptance of the role it has to play. Start by writing, "Dear anxiety, thank you for making me so uncomfortable that I couldn't stay where I was. Thank you for being there to guide me...." Write out all the ways that anxiety has brought wonderful new insights, growth, wisdom, experiences, and positive changes into your life. Without the anxiety making you feel so uncomfortable, would you ever have moved or grown? Feel into gratitude for anxiety now.

Week Twelve Checklist

For the final week, you'll find four powerful practices to have fun with. Read through the full practice guidance for more clarity. And congratulations on reaching Week Twelve!

☐ Consider a bleak or tragic event in your life and open yourself to the possibility of finding something of value in it.

☐ Take a leap of faith. Play with the idea of trusting that you can create something you'd love to experience.

☐ Experiment with creating the expectation that people will be warm and friendly toward you. See what happens.

☐ Write a letter of gratitude to anxiety. Shift into a respectful acceptance of the role it has to play.

Conclusion: Final Words

It is an immense achievement to reach the end of this book. I hope you have applied as many of the practices as you've been able to and that have felt right to you. Take a moment to reflect on how far you have come since you first began. Who was that person before? What was your life like? What kinds of thoughts were you thinking then? What were you feeling? What did you believe? How did you see yourself and the world? How has that shifted for you now?

This process has taken consistency and a real commitment from you. For that, reaching this point of completion, you should be so proud. It is normal to miss bits and not feel resonance with every practice in this book. Do not let the imperfection of your journey through this work take away from celebrating how far you have come. Be proud of yourself. Say those words out loud to yourself now. Bring in your loving parent with arms wrapped around you. It is no easy feat to tackle the issues we encountered together here, to walk into anxiety's fire. Take a moment to sit in reverence for what has burned away and can never come back. I am so proud of you. It has been my honor to write this for you.

Over the last twelve weeks, you have learned:

- You can tune in to your body to find that peaceful perspective of the observer whenever you need to. There is always a place to go to take a holiday from your mind.

- You can build and nurture your mental health resilience. It is not fixed, and you can influence it through the way you take care of yourself.
- You are so much more than an anxious person.

Now you are armed with the tools you need to build your resilience. You can fill in those gaps in your Resilience Shield whenever you feel challenged or knocked by life. When anxiety comes up, you know exactly what you need to do.

In the section following—the Resilience Checklist—you'll find a summary of the steps to follow. You can always come back to your true self, the calm, observing presence, when you feel anxious. Keep this page saved somewhere so you can revisit it easily. With this guidance you'll always know how to figure out what anxiety is telling you and how to respond to its call.

The Resilience Checklist

If you've been feeling stressed and anxious, check in with the areas of your Resilience Shield that require support.

☐ **Awareness of thoughts:** What kinds of thoughts are you thinking? What stories are you telling yourself that need to be rewritten? What scarcity beliefs are challenging you? Do you need to release your emotions? Have you been tuning in to your body? Whose approval are you seeking? Are your thoughts the absolute truth? How can you see the situation with more compassion, love, and forgiveness? What does your inner child need from your loving parent? Are you placing too much emphasis on the worst-case scenario? What if it all goes right? What if there are solutions, possibilities, and opportunities that you can't yet see?

☐ **Connecting to nature:** How much time are you spending in nature? Do you need to spend some time alone in nature?

☐ **Fun, rest, and sleep:** How could you allow yourself to feel more joy? Are you experiencing pleasure in your day-to-day life? How much sleep are you getting at the moment?

☐ **Hormonal balance:** Are you due for your period? Have you been tracking your cycles? Do you need to take supplements to support your progesterone levels?

☐ **Meaningful connections:** What kinds of people are you spending time with? Could you spend more time with loved ones and people who inspire you?

☐ **Movement:** Are you moving your body daily? Could you go for a fifteen-minute walk? Are you exhausting yourself with too much exercise?

☐ **Nutritional needs met:** Are you eating regular meals? Do you need to take any nutritional supplements?

☐ **Optimal gut health:** Are your bowel movements regular? Are you bloating often? Do you have loose stools? Does your gut need some support with bone broth, fiber, and probiotics?

☐ **Prudent use of stimulants:** What is your current level of consumption of alcohol and caffeine (black tea, chocolate, coffee, energy drinks, and so on)? Do you need to make any changes?

Your Lifetime of Healing

While this marks the conclusion of your guided tour through the Anxiety Reset Method, it is not the end of your healing. Mastery is a lifelong process where you'll fall off the horse and get back on count-less times as life's challenges continue to crash at your shores.

Now the rest of your journey begins. It is your responsibility to keep watching that anxious mind, to work on your thoughts and beliefs, to keep showing up for yourself. You can always find support by returning back to the Resilience Checklist, leaning on your journal, and repeating the practices in this book. Should you wish to take this further, you can join in the live experience of my programs, working with me personally.

It is my hope that going forward you can refer back to this book as a helpful guide, but that you also learn to embody and practice the principles of the Anxiety Reset Method—weaving them seamlessly into your life as you need, according to what feels good for you.

Thank you for coming on this journey with me. And thank god for anxiety, bringing us all home to who we truly are.

Resources for Going Deeper

Georgie's Resources

- *The Anxiety Reset Podcast*—A significant audio resource available for free wherever you get your podcasts.
- **The Anxiety Reset Program**—The complete online journey through the Anxiety Reset Method, applying the tools and practices with support.
- **Georgie on Instagram**—You can find me on Instagram here: @georgiethenaturopath.
- **Georgie's website**—To learn more about my latest offerings and events to help you reset your anxious mind, please visit www.georgiecollinson.com.

Life-Changing Books

For general anxiety:

- *Cleaning Up Your Mental Mess*, Dr. Caroline Leaf.
- *First, We Make the Beast Beautiful*, Sarah Wilson.
- *Lost Connections*, Johann Hari.
- *The Wisdom of Anxiety*, Sheryl Paul.

For life advice:

- *Big Magic*, Elizabeth Gilbert.
- *Connected*, Nicholas Christakis and James Fowler.
- *Expectation Hangover*, Christine Hassler.
- *Fearlessly Failing*, Lola Berry.
- *I Am Enough*, Marisa Peer.

For spiritual development:

- *The Power of Now*, Eckhart Tolle.
- *The Tibetan Book of Living and Dying*, Sogyal Rinpoche.
- *You Already Know*, Helen Jacobs.
- *You Can Heal Your Life*, Louise Hay.

For financial anxiety:

- *It's Not Your Money*, Tosha Silver.
- *She's on the Money*, Victoria Devine.

For relationship anxiety:

- *Attached*, Amir Levine and Rachel Heller.

For hormone-based anxiety:

- *Hormone Repair Manual*, Lara Briden.
- *Period Repair Manual*, Lara Briden.

Mental Health Crisis Support

If you're in immediate danger or need urgent assistance, call 911.

If you need to talk to someone about your mental health, you can contact the following services:

- **988 Suicide & Crisis Lifeline:** Dial 988 or visit 988lifeline .org
- **NAMI (National Alliance on Mental Illness):** Dial 1-800-950-6264 or visit www.nami.org/help
- **Substance Abuse and Mental Health Services Administration:** Dial 1-800-662-4357 or visit www.samhsa.gov/find -help/national-helpline

Acknowledgments

We do our best work when we ask for and accept help, and so this book is a culmination of the efforts of many patient, talented, and loving people in my life. A big thank-you to my mother, Jane, my sister, Kate, my cousin Sam, the rest of my family, and my dear friends Steph, Bec, and Laura, all of whom have supported me in countless ways, so I could birth this book to you.

My assistant and friend, also named Steph, has been a tenacious supporter in bringing so many of my projects to life, and for that I am so grateful.

I'd like to express my gratitude to Lola Berry, who has been a fabulous mentor and friend, and to the wonderful Sarah Wilson, who was so kind as to endorse the book with her heartfelt words.

Thank you to my fellow Affirm Press authors, whose support and warmth were the welcome into authorhood of my dreams.

To my community of coaches, healers, podcasters, and therapists, thank you for being the kind of women who support other women, and for adding a little extra magic into my life.

To my friends in Portugal, Australia, Bali, and beyond, thank you for cheering me on every step of the way. You made the process so enjoyable.

To my clients over the years who have trusted me and helped me refine my skills as a healer, allowing me the great honor of providing such fulfilling work, thank you.

Acknowledgments

To the team at Affirm Press (particularly Kelly Doust, Martin Hughes, Keiran Rogers, and Armelle Davies), thank you for believing in my voice and vision for this book, and for giving me the opportunity to share my work with the world. Thank you also to my copyeditor, Brooke Lyons, who tended to my words with such care.

Finally, my dear reader, I am most grateful to you for being brave enough to trust that there can be another way of life for you. May anxiety always serve as a loyal guide, calling you home to your true self.

With love,
Georgie

References

Anxiety in My Life

1. S. Rinpoche, *The Tibetan Book of Living and Dying: The Spiritual Classic and International Bestseller, 30th Anniversary Edition* (San Francisco: HarperSanFrancisco, 2020).

Week One: Tuning In

1. B. M. Wipfli, C. D. Rethorst, and D. M. Landers, "The Anxiolytic Effects of Exercise: A Meta-Analysis of Randomized Trials and Dose-Response Analysis," *Journal of Sport and Exercise Psychology* 30, no. 4 (2008): 392–410.

2. E. Aylett, N. Small, and P. Bower, "Exercise in the Treatment of Clinical Anxiety in General Practice—A Systematic Review and Meta-Analysis," *BMC Health Services Research* 18, no. 1 (2018): 559.

3. K. L. Felmingham, C. Dobson-Stone, P. R. Schofield, G. J. Quirk, and R. A. Bryant, "The Brain-Derived Neurotrophic Factor Val66Met Polymorphism Predicts Response to Exposure Therapy in Posttraumatic Stress Disorder," *Biological Psychiatry* 73, no. 11 (2013): 1059–1063; K. Kobayashi, E. Shimizu, K. Hashimoto, M. Mitsumori, K. Koike, N. Okamura, H. Koizumi, et al., "Serum Brain-Derived Neurotrophic Factor (BDNF) Levels in Patients with Panic Disorder: As a Biological Predictor of Response to Group Cognitive Behavioral Therapy," *Progress in Neuropsychopharmacology & Biological Psychiatry* 29, no. 5 (2005): 658–663.

Week Two: Understanding Anxiety

1. K. M. Jones, L. Brown, E. E. Houston, and C. Bryant, "The Role of Self-Compassion in the Relationship Between Hot Flushes and Night Sweats and Anxiety," *Maturitas* 144 (2021): 81–86.

References

2   W. R. Lovallo, N. H. Farag, A. S. Vincent, T. L. Thomas, and M. F. Wilson, "Cortisol Responses to Mental Stress, Exercise, and Meals Following Caffeine Intake in Men and Women," *Pharmacology, Biochemistry, and Behavior* 83, no. 3 (2006): 441–447.

Week Three: Believing It Can Change

1   N. Rohleder, "Stress and Inflammation—the Need to Address the Gap in the Transition Between Acute and Chronic Stress Effects," *Psychoneuroendocrinology* 105 (2019): 164–171.

2   V. Magnon, F. Dutheil, and G. T. Vallet, "Benefits from One Session of Deep and Slow Breathing on Vagal Tone and Anxiety in Young and Older Adults," *Scientific Reports* 11, no. 1 (2021): 1–10.

3   H. B. Rankhambe and S. Pande, "Effect of 'Om' Chanting on Anxiety in Bus Drivers," *National Journal of Physiology, Pharmacy and Pharmacology* 10, no. 12 (2020): 1138–1141.

4   M. D. Dogan, "The Effect of Laughter Therapy on Anxiety: A Meta-Analysis," *Holistic Nursing Practice* 34, no. 1 (2020): 35–39.

Week Four: Uncovering the Truth

1   S. Banskota, J. E. Ghia, and W. I. Khan, "Serotonin in the Gut: Blessing or a Curse," *Biochimie* 161 (2019): 56–64.

2   G. Agirman, K. B. Yu, and E. Y. Hsiao, "Signaling Inflammation Across the Gut–Brain Axis," *Science* 374, no. 6571 (2021): 1087–1092.

3   A. Fasano, "All Disease Begins in the (Leaky) Gut: Role of Zonulin-Mediated Gut Permeability in the Pathogenesis of Some Chronic Inflammatory Diseases," *F1000Research* 9 (2020).

4   F. Mei, Z. Duan, M. Chen, J. Lu, M. Zhao, L. Li, X. Shen, G. Xia, and S. Chen, "Effect of a High-Collagen Peptide Diet on the Gut Microbiota and Short-Chain Fatty Acid Metabolism," *Journal of Functional Foods* 75 (2020): 104278.

5   B. J. Deters and M. Saleem, "The Role of Glutamine in Supporting Gut Health and Neuropsychiatric Factors," *Food Science and Human Wellness* 10, no. 2 (2021): 149–154.

6   A. L. Lopresti, "The Problem of Curcumin and Its Bioavailability: Could Its Gastrointestinal Influence Contribute to Its Overall Health-Enhancing Effects?," *Advances in Nutrition* 9, no. 1 (2018): 41–50.

References

Week Six: Making Miracles

1 M. Rostami-Nejad, N. Taraghikhah, C. Ciacci, M. A. Pourhoseingholi, F. Barzegar, M. Rezaei-Tavirani, D. Aldulaimi, and M. R. Zali, "Anxiety Symptoms in Adult Celiac Patients and the Effect of a Gluten-Free Diet: An Iranian Nationwide Study," *Inflammatory Intestinal Diseases* 5, no. 1 (2020): 42–47.

2 G. Caio, L. Lungaro, N. Segata, M. Guarino, G. Zoli, U. Volta, and R. De Giorgio, "Effect of Gluten-Free Diet on Gut Microbiota Composition in Patients with Celiac Disease and Non-Celiac Gluten/Wheat Sensitivity," *Nutrients* 12, no. 6 (2020): 1832.

3 J. Kose, A. Cheung, L. K. Fezeu, S. Péneau, C. Debras, M. Touvier, S. Hercberg, P. Galan, and V. A. Andreeva, "A Comparison of Sugar Intake Between Individuals with High and Low Trait Anxiety: Results from the NutriNet-Santé Study," *Nutrients* 13, no. 5 (2021): 1526.

4 B. Mahdavifar, M. Hosseinzadeh, A. Salehi-Abargouei, M. Mirzaei, and M. Vafa, "The Association between Dairy Products and Psychological Disorders in a Large Sample of Iranian Adults," *Nutritional Neuroscience* 25, no. 11 (2022): 2379–2389.

5 O. Sadeghi, A. H. Keshteli, H. Afshar, A. Esmaillzadeh, and P. Adibi, "Adherence to Mediterranean Dietary Pattern Is Inversely Associated with Depression, Anxiety and Psychological Distress," *Nutritional Neuroscience* 24, no. 4 (2021): 248–259; A. Ventriglio, F. Sancassiani, M. P. Contu, M. Latorre, M. Di Slavatore, M. Fornaro, and D. Bhugra, "Mediterranean Diet and Its Benefits on Health and Mental Health: A Literature Review," *Clinical Practice and Epidemiology in Mental Health* 16, Suppl-1 (2020): 156–164.

6 U. Dobersek, G. Wy, J. Adkins, S. Altmeyer, K. Krout, C. J. Lavie, and E. Archer, "Meat and Mental Health: A Systematic Review of Meat Abstention and Depression, Anxiety, and Related Phenomena," *Critical Reviews in Food Science and Nutrition* 61, no. 4 (2021): 622–635.

7 P. M. Kris-Etherton, K. S. Petersen, J. R. Hibbeln, D. Hurley, V. Kolick, S. Peoples, N. Rodriguez, and G. Woodward-Lopez, "Nutrition and Behavioral Health Disorders: Depression and Anxiety," *Nutrition Reviews* 79, no. 3 (2021): 247–260.

Week Seven: Pleasure

1 R. L. Roberts, J. R. Rhodes, and G. R. Elkins, "Effect of Hypnosis on Anxiety: Results from a Randomized Controlled Trial with Women in Postmenopause," *Journal of Clinical Psychology in Medical Settings* 28, no. 4 (2021): 868–881.

References

Week Eight: A Bright Future

1   L. S. LaFreniere and M. G. Newman, "Exposing Worry's Deceit: Percentage of Untrue Worries in Generalized Anxiety Disorder Treatment," *Behavior Therapy* 51, no. 3 (2020): 413–423.

2   K. Savage, J. Firth, C. Stough, and J. Sarris, "GABA-Modulating Phytomedicines for Anxiety: A Systematic Review of Preclinical and Clinical Evidence," *Phytotherapy Research* 32, no. 1 (2018): 3–18.

Week Nine: Nurture with Nature

1   Y. Kotera, M. Lyons, K. C. Vione, and B. Norton, "Effect of Nature Walks on Depression and Anxiety: A Systematic Review," *Sustainability* 13, no. 7 (2021): 4015.

2   G. N. Bratman, J. P. Hamilton, K. S. Hahn, G. C. Daily, and J. J. Gross, "Nature Experience Reduces Rumination and Subgenual Prefrontal Cortex Activation," *Proceedings of the National Academy of Sciences* 112, no. 28 (2015): 8567–8572.

3   Y. Kotera, M. Richardson, and D. Sheffield, "Effects of Shinrin-Yoku (Forest Bathing) and Nature Therapy on Mental Health: A Systematic Review and Meta-Analysis," *International Journal of Mental Health and Addiction* 20, no. 1 (2022): 337–361.

4   E. Bielinis, N. Takayama, S. Boiko, A. Omelan, and L. Bielinis, "The Effect of Winter Forest Bathing on Psychological Relaxation of Young Polish Adults," *Urban Forestry & Urban Greening* 29 (2018): 276–283; M. R. Hunter, B. W. Gillespie, and S. Y. P. Chen, "Urban Nature Experiences Reduce Stress in the Context of Daily Life Based on Salivary Biomarkers," *Frontiers in Psychology* 10 (2019): 722.

5   Hunter, Gillespie, and Chen, "Urban Nature Experiences Reduce Stress in the Context of Daily Life Based on Salivary Biomarkers."

6   L. Martin, M. P. White, A. Hunt, M. Richardson, S. Pahl, and J. Burt, "Nature Contact, Nature Connectedness and Associations with Health, Wellbeing and Pro-Environmental Behaviours," *Journal of Environmental Psychology* 68 (2020): 101389.

7   J. Nguyen and E. Brymer, "Nature-Based Guided Imagery as an Intervention for State Anxiety," *Frontiers in Psychology* 9 (2018): 1858.

8   J. Kim and M. Wessling-Resnick, "Iron and Mechanisms of Emotional Behavior," *Journal of Nutritional Biochemistry* 25, no. 11 (2014): 1101–1107.

9   E. N. G. Buita, D. A. R. Castor, E. S. Condat, M. L. E. Cuaderno, J. M. G. Cunan, F. A. V. Danao, M. L. Daya, and V. G. Villegas, "Association of Symptoms-Based Iron Deficiency Anemia to Anxiety and Depression Related Criteria Symptoms Among the 3rd Year Medical Technology Students of the University of Santo Tomas During the COVID-19 Pandemic," *International Journal of Progressive Research in Science and Engineering* 2, no. 10 (2021): 62–71.

10 H. S. Lee, H. H. Chao, W. T. Huang, S. C. C. Chen, and H. Y. Yang, "Psychiatric Disorders Risk in Patients with Iron Deficiency Anemia and Association with Iron Supplementation Medications: A Nationwide Database Analysis," *BMC Psychiatry* 20, no. 1 (2020): 216.

Week Ten: The External World

1   N. A. Christakis and J. H. Fowler, *Connected: The Surprising Power of Our Social Networks and How They Shape Our Lives—How Your Friends' Friends' Friends Affect Everything You Feel, Think, and Do* (New York: Little, Brown Spark, 2011).

2   F. Kader, M. Ghai, and L. Maharaj, "The Effects of DNA Methylation on Human Psychology," *Behavioural Brain Research* 346 (2018): 47–65.

3   Kader, Ghai, and Maharaj, "The Effects of DNA Methylation on Human Psychology."

4   S. Moll and E. A. Varga, "Homocysteine and MTHFR Mutations," *Circulation* 132, no. 1 (2015): e6–e9.

5   M. Rainka, J. Meaney, E. Westphal, T. S. Aladeen, K. M. Landolf, S. B. Stanford, P. Galdun, N. Asbach, F. Gengo, and H. Capote, "Effect of L-methylfolate on Depressive Symptoms in Patients with MTHFR Mutations (P3.9-057)," *Neurology* 92 (2019).

Week Eleven: Healthy Emotional Expression

1   J. Zhang, X. Zhang, K. Zhang, X. Lu, G. Yuan, H. Yang, H. Guo, et al., "An Updated of Meta-Analysis on the Relationship Between Mobile Phone Addiction and Sleep Disorder," *Journal of Affective Disorders* 305 (2022): 94–101.

2   H. H. Lin, P. S. Tsai, S. C. Fang, and J. F. Liu, "Effect of Kiwifruit Consumption on Sleep Quality in Adults with Sleep Problems," *Asia Pacific Journal of Clinical Nutrition* 20, no. 2 (2011): 169–174.

References

3   A. L. Hansen, L. Dahl, G. Olson, D. Thornton, I. E. Graff, L. Frøyland, J. F. Thayer, and S. Pallesen, "Fish Consumption, Sleep, Daily Functioning, and Heart Rate Variability," *Journal of Clinical Sleep Medicine* 10, no. 5 (2014): 567–575.

4   G. Howatson, P. G. Bell, J. Tallent, B. Middleton, M. P. McHugh, and J. Ellis, "Effect of Tart Cherry Juice (Prunus cerasus) on Melatonin Levels and Enhanced Sleep Quality," *European Journal of Nutrition* 51, no. 8 (2012): 909–916.

About the Author

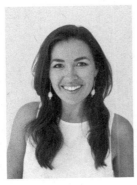

Georgie Collinson is an anxiety mindset coach, hypnotherapist, and degree-qualified nutritionist and naturopath. As a recovering perfectionist and proud high achiever, Georgie was once the prime example of someone with high-functioning anxiety. Searching for answers, she discovered a lasting breakthrough for herself and her clients: a holistic mind–body approach that considers anxiety and stress arising from thoughts, food, gut health, hormones, and lifestyle. She developed this into the Anxiety Reset® Method, and her successful online Anxiety Reset Program. Georgie is known for her vulnerable, honest, and down-to-earth way of speaking about mental health. She hosts the *Anxiety Reset Podcast* and has appeared on live national television, guest blogs, and in numerous podcast interviews. Originally from Melbourne, Australia, Georgie is based on Victoria's Mornington Peninsula and coaches clients from all over the world.